André Gustavo Fernandes de Oliveira
Marcelo F. Costa
Dora Fix Ventura

Visual Development

André Gustavo Fernandes de Oliveira
Marcelo F. Costa
Dora Fix Ventura

Visual Development

Acuity functions and contrast sensitivity in babies

ScienciaScripts

Imprint
Any brand names and product names mentioned in this book are subject to trademark, brand or patent protection and are trademarks or registered trademarks of their respective holders. The use of brand names, product names, common names, trade names, product descriptions etc. even without a particular marking in this work is in no way to be construed to mean that such names may be regarded as unrestricted in respect of trademark and brand protection legislation and could thus be used by anyone.

Cover image: www.ingimage.com

This book is a translation from the original published under ISBN 978-3-330-77107-9.

Publisher:
Sciencia Scripts
is a trademark of
Dodo Books Indian Ocean Ltd. and OmniScriptum S.R.L publishing group

120 High Road, East Finchley, London, N2 9ED, United Kingdom
Str. Armeneasca 28/1, office 1, Chisinau MD-2012, Republic of Moldova, Europe
Managing Directors: Ieva Konstantinova, Victoria Ursu
info@omniscriptum.com

Printed at: see last page
ISBN: 978-620-8-63551-0

index:

Thanks

To my dear parents, Humberto and Vânia, who with great effort made this work possible;

To my aunt and uncle, Liomério and Nélia, for welcoming me to Sao Paulo and making me one of their own, and to my cousin Bruno, a brother in Sao Paulo;

To my wife Flàvia, who encourages me to pursue my greatest goals;

To my daughters Marcela and Isadora, the cover models and treasures of my life;

To my tutors, professors and lab colleagues, for the constant opportunity to learn and collaborate;

To FAPESP, for the support granted under processes 03/10342-4 and 05/60064-6.

To the Participants and Responsible Persons who took part in the research, because without them there is no science!

Summary

The development of the nervous system is extremely complex and, if analyzed in detail, can be described as fascinating. One of the strategies for this analysis includes assessing the visual system. It is well known that the visual world of a newborn is considerably different and very impoverished compared to that of an adult. Basic visual functions such as visual acuity and contrast sensitivity are immature at birth, but undergo major changes during childhood. The visual development of a baby born prematurely is even more curious. Prematurity at birth is a risk factor for vision, and we don't know if babies, even with apparently normal visual development, actually follow the same course as that observed in babies born after a full gestation, or if they also suffer some damage due to premature birth. Alternatively, these babies could have accelerated visual development due to their longer exposure to the visual world. In order to find out whether the condition of prematurity accelerates, delays or does not alter the development of vision, this book compares the development of visual acuity and spatial luminance contrast sensitivity functions in babies born prematurely and at term. The research methods include Provoked Cortical Visual Potential Scans, and possible correlations between visual thresholds obtained during the first year of life and gestational age, Apgar scores, and birth weight values are also examined.

I - Introduction

I . 1 - Prematurity

The current concept of prematurity was defined in 1969 by the *World Health Organization (WHO).* Any live newborn child with less than 37 weeks of gestation or 259 days (WHO, 1970) counted from the first day of the last menstrual period is considered premature (Rades, Bittar & Zugaib, 2004).

While in the last decade we have seen an improvement in birth standards including improvements in the quality of pre- and perinatal care (Spallicci et al., 2000), a decrease in the number of women who smoke during pregnancy, and a decrease in the number of deliveries by caesarean section, the prevalence of preterm births has been increasing steadily since 1976 (Birch & O'Connor, 2001). This increase is associated with the rise in the prevalence of multiple births as well as with changes in maternal characteristics which include a greater number of mothers over 35 years of age, a greater number of mothers who have had successful high-risk pregnancies, as well as a greater number of extremely young mothers (Birch & O'Connor, 2001).

The incidence of prematurity is variable, depending on population characteristics, and has generally increased every year except in some countries such as France and Finland (Rades, Bittar & Zugaib, 2004). A study carried out in the United States in 1997 revealed an incidence of 11.3% of premature births that year - 0.1% more than the previous year - and an incidence of 7.5% of low birth weight births, with an increase over the previous year of 0.1% equal to that of gestational age. During the period from 1981 to 2003, there was a 27% increase in the incidence of prematurity in the United States (Rades, Bittar & Zugaib, 2004).

In Brazil, information on premature births is scarcer and less reliable, according to Rades, Bittar & Zugaib (2004). The work of Spallicci et al. (2000) reveals an incidence ranging from 5 to 15%. The SEADE Foundation (State Data Analysis System) recorded 7.07% of premature births in the city of São Paulo in 2001, unlike the Obstetrics Clinic of the HCFMUSP (Hospital das Clinicas of the Faculty of Medicine of the University of São Paulo) which recorded an average incidence of prematurity of 22% between 1993 and 2002 (Rades, Bittar & Zugaib, 2004). The large discrepancy in this data can be explained by the fact that HCFMUSP is classified as a tertiary hospital.

An important health condition for newborns is their size, and consequently their weight. Premature newborns are often small for their gestational age. The term "small for gestational age" (SGA) describes a child whose birth weight in relation to gestational age is below a pre-determined cut-off point, which varies from study to study, and there is a direct relationship between the difference in weight in relation to gestational age and the increased incidence of health problems (Ornelas, Xavier & Colosimo, 2002). The performance of small-for-gestational-age premature newborns in terms of their growth and development, in addition to their genetic potential, depends on the quality of medical and hospital care and, after discharge, on the family's socio-economic conditions (Ornelas, Xavier & Colosimo, 2002).

Premature birth can be classified according to different parameters, including birth weight, gestational age, Apgar score or even the etiology of prematurity, as described by Moutquin (2003).

The etiological factors of premature birth are spontaneous birth, caused by spontaneous labor or premature rupture of membranes, and elective birth, by medical indication, due to maternal and/or fetal complications (Rades, Bittar & Zugaib, 2004).

Despite advances in perinatology in recent years, premature birth continues to be the main cause of neonatal morbidity and mortality, representing one of the greatest challenges for obstetrics (Birch & O'Connor, 2001; Mazzitelli, 2002; Rades, Bittar & Zugaib, 2004). Around 75% of newborn deaths in this period were due to prematurity, excluding malformations, while morbidity is directly related to respiratory disorders and infectious and neurological complications, as described in the study by Rades, Bittar & Zugaib (2004).

Premature birth potentially represents an important factor in visual development, acting in two different ways (Birch & O' Connor, 2001). According to these authors, firstly, premature exteriorization subjects the visual system to early visual stimulation and simultaneously deprives it of essential nutrients transferred from the mother to the fetus via the placenta during the final phase of pregnancy, a period of rapid maturation of this system. Secondly, immaturity, together with the various associations and systemic complications of premature birth, places the child in a risk group for permanent visual alterations (Birch & O'Connor, 2001).

According to Egyetem & Klinika (1999) the most characteristic illness found in premature infants is Idiopathic Respiratory Distress Syndrome. Problems related to vision, hearing and neurological development are integral parts of neonatal concerns.

Parmelee (1975) reported that some premature infants may indeed be advanced in various areas of behavior and neurophysiological development, but this is counterbalanced by premature infants who are significantly impaired in these parameters for medical reasons such as hypoxia or metabolic disorders, while a third of these children show disorganized mixtures of impairments and developmental advances in select areas.

Retinopathy of prematurity is caused by an alteration in the interaction between the cells that make up the retina during development. The retina, as part of the nervous system, contains neurons, glial cells (astrocytes and Muller cells) and blood vessels (containing vascular endothelial cells, pericytes, and smooth muscle cells), as well as cells of the immune system and phagocytes. The process of forming the vascularization of the human retina involves complex interactions between these cellular elements in order to produce a vascular network adjusted to the metabolic needs of the tissue (Lutty et al., 2006). During this period, the appearance of retinopathy of prematurity (ROP), a proliferative vascular disease that occurs in premature newborns, is very common. In these babies, at birth, retinal vasculogenesis is incomplete, favoring the formation of neovascular tissue, which in the vast majority of cases involutes spontaneously. However, in a minority of cases, it develops into fibrovascular proliferation towards the vitreous, forming retinal membranes and traces, which can lead to retinal detachment and poor visual resolution in these eyes (Bonotto, Moreira & Carvalho, 2007). One third of children born weighing less than 1,500g may have ROP, and this incidence increases to 65.8% when the birth weight is less than 1,250g and 81.6% when it is less than 1,000g. Blindness is a consequence of PON in 0.5% of babies born weighing between 1000 and 1500g, as well as scarring which occurs in 2.2% of babies born in this weight range (Dambro, 2002).

Multicenter studies indicate that the peripheral production of growth factors in the avascular retina may be the probable disorder that leads to retinal deterioration in ROP processes (Lutty et al., 2006).

Various etiological factors have been associated with the development of POP, such as low birth weight and gestational age, infections, vitamin E and A deficiency, as well as excessive exposure to light (Bonotto, Moreira & Carvalho, 2007).

A higher incidence of visual alterations in premature infants with and without a diagnosis of ROP compared to term newborns is widely described in the literature (Birch & O'Connor, 2001; Haro, 2003; Jongmans et al., 1996; Kos-Pietro et al., 1997; Lutty et al., 2006; Mash & Dobson, 1998; Mazzitelli, 2002; Norcia Tyler and Hamer, 1990; Pike et al., 1994; Salomao et al., 2001).

Results of studies by the *CRYO-ROP Cooperative* group, which studies the treatment of ROP with cryotherapy techniques, show benefits of this technique in the development of VA when applied to eyes with severe retinopathy. This does not exclude the need for methods to prevent the development of retinopathy or the need to improve the techniques that can treat this pathology (Lutty et al., 2006).

I . 2 - Visual Acuity and Contrast Sensitivity

The visual world of a newborn is considerably different and very impoverished compared to that of an adult. Basic visual functions such as visual acuity (VA), contrast sensitivity (CS), stereopsis, color vision, eye movements and oculomotor control are immature at birth, but all these visual capacities undergo great development during infancy, especially in the first months of life (Atkinson & Braddick, 1989; Slater, 1989; Boothe et al.., 1988; Salomao & Ventura 1995, Hamer et al, 1989; Birch & O'Connor 2001; Teller, 1990; Norcia & Tyler, 1985; Van Hof-van Duin & Mohn, 1986).

The most common procedure used in ophthalmology to measure the efficiency of the visual system is the VA test (Atkinson & Braddick, 1989; Cinoto et al., 2006; Odom, 2003). VA at birth is so poor (approximately 20/400 in electrophysiological measurements according to Mills, 1999) that an adult with the VA level of a newborn is legally considered blind (Slater, 1989).

VA can be defined as the visual function that expresses the ability to discriminate shapes. It refers to the measurement of the angular separation threshold between two points in space or the visual resolution of their respective images on the retina (Bicas, 2002).

Visual acuity refers to the spatial limit of visual discrimination. It therefore involves determining a threshold. Within this general definition, we can divide visual acuity into 3 main assessment criteria:

Minimally visible: the ability to detect the presence of a visual stimulus, i.e. the smallest stimulus that can be seen by the subject.

Minimal resolvable: the ability to detect the shortest distance between two stimuli. In a normal adult, the resolution limit, often presented as the angle of minimum resolution (AMR), is between 30 seconds and one minute of arc.

Minimum discriminability: ability to detect spatial differences when the threshold is below the minimum separability, i.e. within a few seconds of arc.

Factors such as optical aberrations, refractive errors, diffractions that occur at the edge of the pupil and the pupil size itself, the modulation transfer function of the optical system and the visual pathway, luminance, retinal eccentricity of the image and the distance between the photoreceptors all influence visual acuity (Hart, 1992).

For conventional clinical AV measurement, visual characters called optotypes are presented to the patient, who is asked to identify them. The optotypes are usually presented at a very high contrast, and as correct identification answers are obtained, the size of the optotypes is gradually reduced (the details become finer) until the patient makes a mistake or reports that they cannot identify the optotype. The VA corresponds to the smallest optotype identified and is a measure of the visual system's greatest resolving capacity (Schwartz, 2004).

VA is usually determined using printed tables with the Snellen Optotypes. Other testing methodologies, such as computerized programs using "E" optotypes, have also been scientifically proven to be effective tools for assessing VA, providing objective results, with the advantage of independence from the examiner's interaction during the test (Beck et al., 2003; Arippol, Salomao & Belfort Jr., 2006).

AV can be measured through different tasks:

- **Detection task:** consists of detecting the presence or absence of some aspect of the visual stimulus, without the need to report details about the stimulus, as shown in figure 1. The acuity measured is the minimum visible.

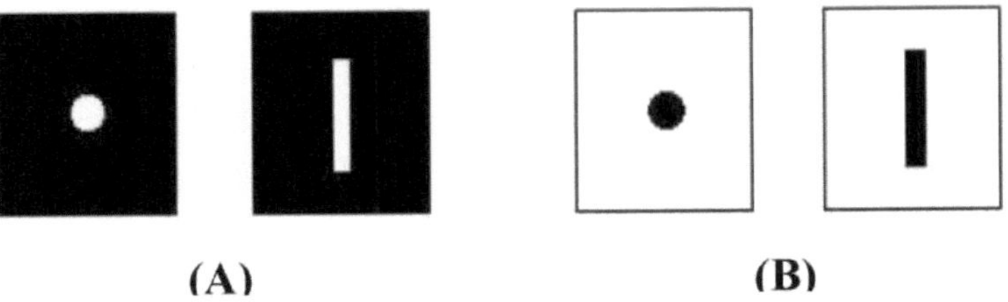

Fig. 1 - The detection task involves determining the presence of a dot or a line. (A) Light test object on a dark background. (B) Dark test object on a light background.

(Kolb et al., 2007) webvision.med.utah.edu/KallSpatiaLhtml

▪ **Recognition task:** consists of recognizing or naming an optotype, and therefore requires these test optotypes to be larger than the subject's detection limit (figure 2). The acuity measured is the minimum resolvable.

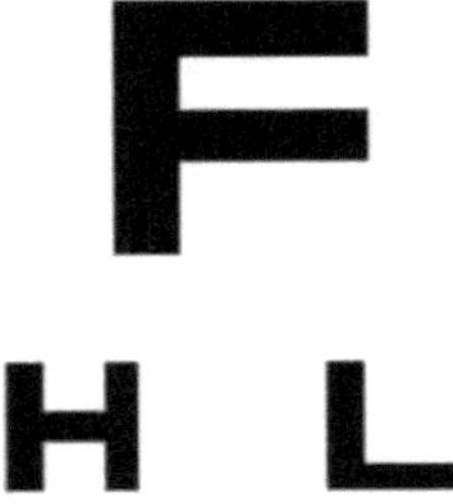

Fig. 2 - Recognition task. Naming the test object, in this case the letters of the Alphabet (Snellen).

(Kolb et al., 2007webvision.med.utah.edu/KallSpatial.html

The *non-literal E and Landolt's C* are two more common forms of AV measures (optotypes) used clinically through recognition tasks. In these cases, exemplified in figure 3, the task is to recognize the positioning of the optotype through the position of the opening (gap) in the stimuli.

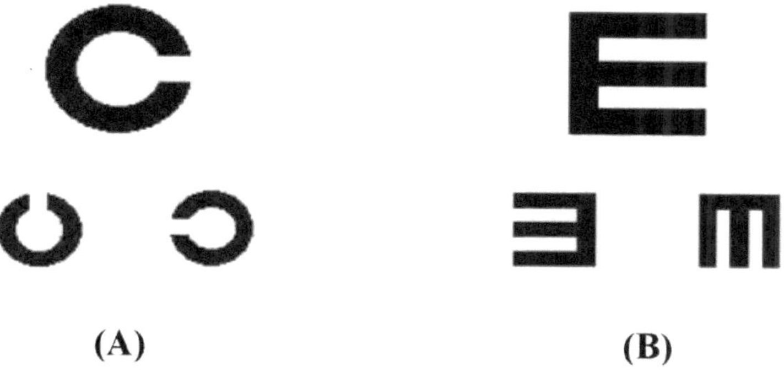

Fig. 3 - (A) *Landolt's C.* (B) *Non-literary E.*

(Kolb et al., 2007**webvision.med.utah.edu/KallSpatial.html**

▪ **Localization task:** consists of discriminating differences in the spatial position of the segments of the test object, such as an interruption or discontinuity of its contour. The acuity measured is the minimum discriminable. Also called Vernier Acuity, it represents a type of hyperacuity. Figure 4 shows examples of stimuli for this type of task.

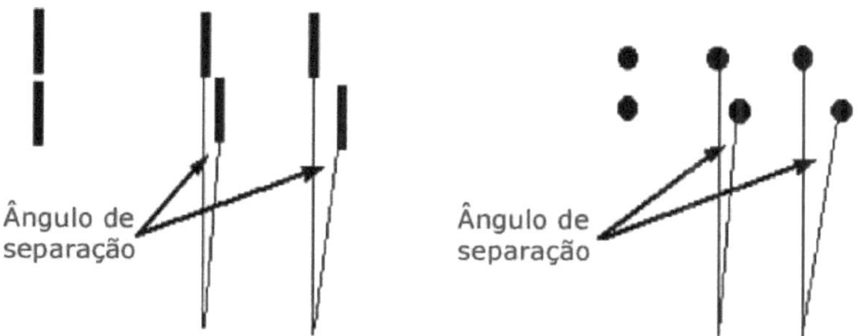

Fig. 4 - Localization task in which the misalignment between stimuli is measured. Examples of stimuli used to measure Vernier Acuity.

(Kolb et al., 2007**webvision.med.utah.edu/KallSpatial.html**

▪ **Resolution threshold task:** this threshold corresponds to the smallest angular size at which a subject can discriminate the separation between critical elements of a standardized stimulus composed of pairs of dots, grids, or squares (figure 5). The acuity measured is the minimum resolvable.

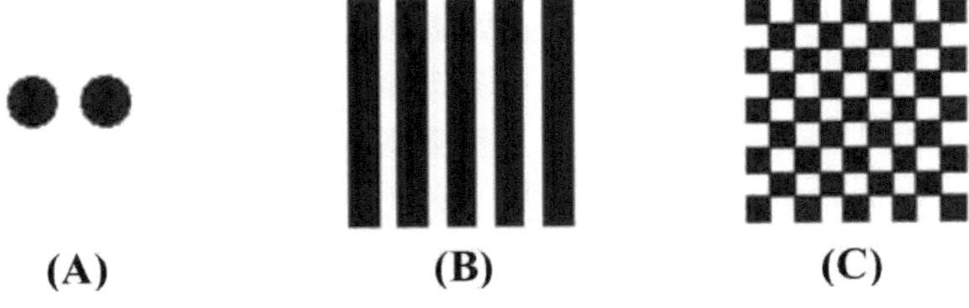

Fig. 5 - Solving task. (A) Pair of dots. (B) Grids. (C) Charts. (Kolb et al., 2007**webvision.med.utah.edu/KallSpatial.html**

Using a grid as a stimulus for AV assessment, for example, the spatial frequency of the grid can be expressed in cycles per degree (cpg) of visual angle, where a cycle consists of a light band and a dark band on the grid (Cornsweet, 1970) (figure 6). Visual angle is the angle formed by an object that is projected onto the retina. This angle relates the width (l) of the object to its distance (d) from the observer. The relationship Visual angle = (l/d) radians, can be expressed in degrees.

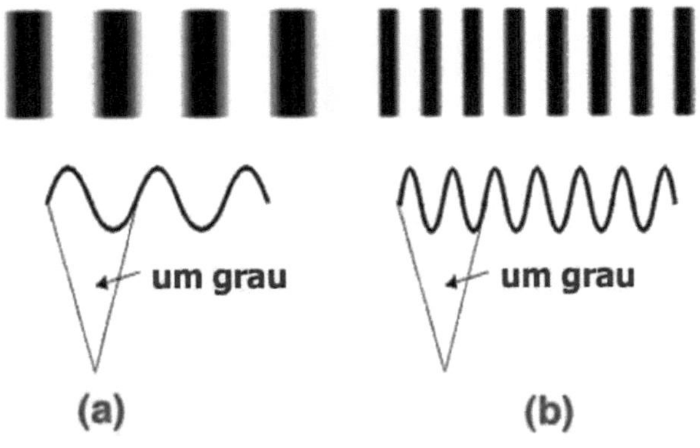

Fig. 6 - Spatial frequency is the measure of the number of cycles per degree Understood on the retina. (a) One cycle per degree. (b) Two cycles per degree.

(Kolb et al., 2007**webvision.med.utah.edu/KallSpatial.html**

Vertical square wave luminance grids were used to measure the resolution threshold in the AV evaluations in this study.

Functionally, a newborn's VA values can be observed from two different perspectives. If on the one hand the VA in the first few months is very low compared to adult values of 30 to 40 cpg, on the other hand the proximity of objects with which newborns primarily relate, such as faces, for example, generates large retinal images and the essence of this information can be made available even with an average VA of just 1 cpg. Therefore, important visual information in the first months of life is probably not limited by acuity, although these limitations contribute to a lack of interest in distant objects, whose retinal images are obviously much smaller (Atkinson & Braddick, 1989).

VA describes the behavior of the visual system in resolving details of a spatial stimulus. However, a more complete measure of human spatial vision comprises the measure of Contrast Sensitivity (CS) (Adams & Courage 2002; Atkinson, Braddick & Braddick, 1974; Atkinson & Braddick, 1989; Campbell, 1974).

CS is one of the most important functions of the visual system in humans and other animals (Shapley, Kaplan, & Purpura, 1993) because it enables us to identify objects. Without the ability to perceive contrasts, we wouldn't be able to see shapes. The greater this ability, the greater the possibility of detecting small variations in the field of vision. The contrast threshold is the smallest detectable difference in luminance or color between two areas juxtaposed spatially or successively in time. Spatial CS is often measured using sinusoidal gratings of different spatial frequencies. In this situation, CS is defined as the reciprocal of the minimum amount of contrast required to detect a grating of a specific spatial frequency (Cornsweet, 1970).

Two surfaces can be perceived as separate if there is a difference in some physical attribute. The difference in luminance between adjacent areas (Campbell, 1974) is a physical property of the visual stimulus, as well as differences in texture, color or others (Cornsweet, 1970; Shapley, Kaplan, & Purpura, 1993).

The luminance contrast can be calculated by measuring the luminances of the surfaces to be compared. In the case of an area in a homogeneous field, Weber's Contrast is used:

$$C_W = L - L_F / L_F,$$

where L is the luminance of the area to be discriminated and LF is the luminance of the background in which that area is located.

For patterns in which lighter and darker areas are approximately equivalent, as occurs in periodic spatials such as sinusoidal grids, the definition of contrast used is:

$$C_R = (L_{max} - L_{min}) / (L_{max} + L_{min})$$

where L_{max} is the maximum luminance and L_{min} the minimum luminance. CR or Rayleigh Contrast (CR) can have absolute values between 0.0 and 1.0, and can also be called Modulation, or Michelson (figure

7) (Shapley, Kaplan, & Purpura, 1993).

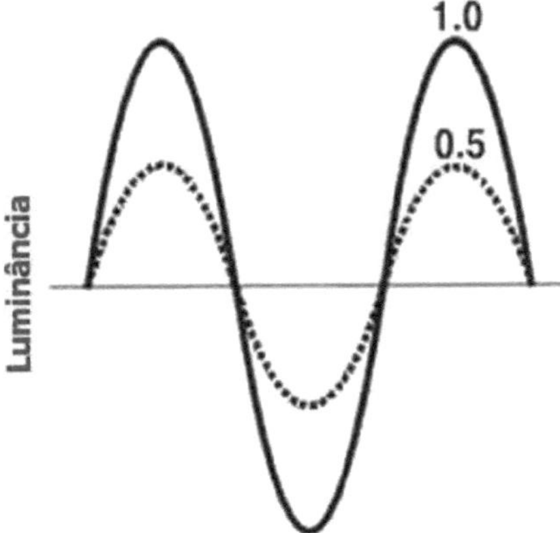

Fig. 7 - Contrast luminance profile of sinusoidal grids in a ratio of 1.0 and 0.5 (Michelson contrast). For a contrast value of 1.0, the grid must have the maximum and minimum luminance available.

(Kolb et al., 2007**webvision.med.utah.edu/KallSpatial.html**

According to Campbell (1974), in the concept that the visual system analyzes a spatial frequency in terms of the simple sum of the harmonics of this frequency, the first step is to study the responses of this system to simple sinusoidal gratings. In this way we can later understand how the visual system deals with more complex waveforms. Following this line of reasoning, for an evaluation of CS, stimuli in the form of sinusoidal or square gratings (stripes) are used as a way of measuring the resolving power of the eye, as they can be adjusted to any spatial frequency providing easily quantifiable results within a Fourier analysis treatment of the spatial pattern (Cornsweet, 1970).

A sinusoidal luminance grating is defined in terms of the modulation of the contrast amplitude and the spatial frequency.

For a complete description of a sine wave grating, in addition to contrast and spatial frequency, the phase and orientation of the grating are important. Phase refers to the position of the sine wave grating in relation to another sine wave grating, whereby if two identical sine wave gratings are in phase, their luminances complement each other, and if these same two gratings are in counter-phase by 1 80 degrees, the peaks and valleys cancel each other out. Orientation refers to the description of the angle corresponding to the gratings (Shapley, Kaplan, & Purpura, 1993).

Most of the studies that have attempted to estimate CS to date have used vertical sinusoidal grids as a standard (Allen, Tyler, & Norcia, 1996; Bradley & Freeman, 1982; de Faria et al., 1998; Hammarrenger et al, 2007; Jackson et al., 2003; Mirabella et al., 2006; Norcia et al., 1989; Norcia, Tyler, & Hamer, 1990; Oliveira et al., 2004; Peterzell & Norcia, 1997; Santos & Simas, 2001;

Shannon, Skoczenski, & Banks, 1996).

The contrast value required by the visual system to reach a threshold can be expressed on a scale of decibels (dB) or as a percentage (%) of contrast. The reciprocal of this value is contrast sensitivity.

Contrast thresholds can be measured at various spatial frequencies. The relationship obtained between contrast amplitude and spatial frequency constitutes the spatial Contrast Sensitivity Function (CSF).

The visual system is more sensitive to some spatial frequencies than others (Atkinson & Braddick, 1989; Campbell, 1974). Under conditions of photopic vision, measuring CS with sinusoidal gratings reveals a band-pass function, i.e. there is a reduction in contrast sensitivity at high and low spatial frequencies (Schwartz, 2004). The cut-off frequency at the high end corresponds to AV, i.e. the spatial frequency at which the maximum contrast is required to detect the smallest possible object at a given average luminance level.

CS was assessed in adults by psychophysical and electrophysiological methods, using the visual-evoked potential scan, at spatial frequencies of 0.5, 1.0, 2.0, 4.0 and 8.0 cpg, by de Faria et al. (1998), and the results showed the best sensitivity at a mean spatial frequency of 2.0 cpg.

At first it is surprising that after an optimal size, as the gratings become larger, the CS becomes smaller until a limit is reached and the gratings are no longer perceived (Campbell, 1974). The explanation for this cut-off of low spatial frequencies is given by the phenomenon of spatial opacity, which results from the action of the lateral inhibition mechanism in the retina. The receptive field of a retinal ganglion cell consists of a central region that responds to light stimuli with excitation or inhibition, and a peripheral region that responds with a signal opposite to that of the central region. As the grid is made up of light and dark bands, a very wide dark or light band (low spatial frequency) is capable of simultaneously activating the central and peripheral regions of the receptive field, nullifying the response to the stimulus (Schwartz, 2004).

The reduction in CS at high spatial frequencies reflects the limitation of the visual system in resolving details, even at 100% contrast (Schwartz, 2004). This limitation reflects the optical properties of the eye, whose resolution is tuned to the mosaic of photoreceptors in the retina. In figure 8 the maximum point of resolution can be seen between 10 and 100 cpg, around 60 cpg, where the FSC crosses the abscissa axis (Kolb et al., 2007).

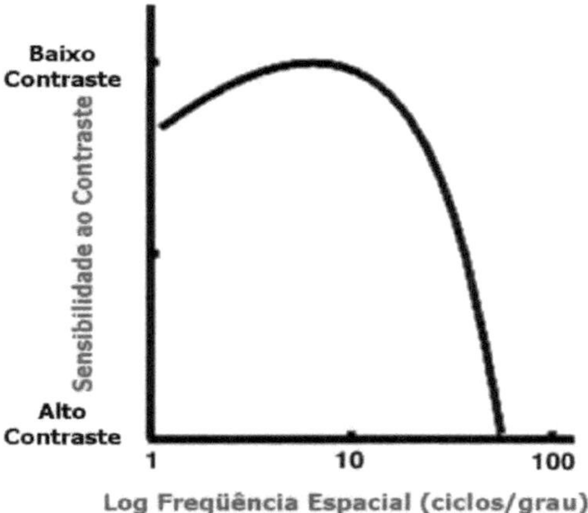

Fig. 8 - Photopic contrast sensitivity function.

(Kolb et al., 2007webvision.med.utah.edu/KallSpatial.html

The better human resolution for intermediate spatial frequencies can also be seen in figure 9, which reproduces figure 8 in a similar way, using grids with spatial frequencies that increase from left to right and with contrast levels that increase from top to bottom in the figure.

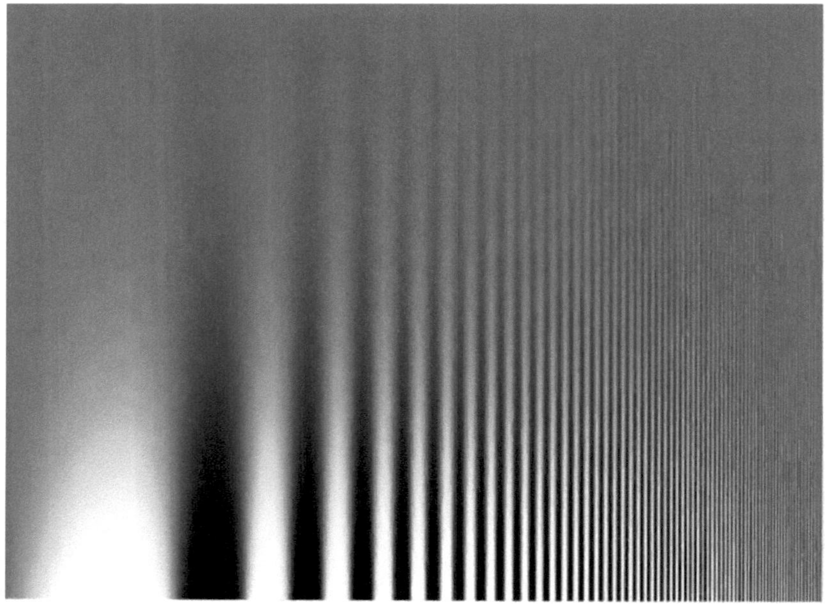

Fig. 9 - Plate showing FSC. The contrast increases from the top to the bottom of the figure, and the spatial frequency increases from left to right (Ohzawa, I. 2007).

http://cobalt056.bpe.es.osaka-u.ac.jP/ohzawa-lab/izumi/CSF/A JG RobsonCSFcharLhtml

The shape and critical parameters of the FSC depend on a number of factors including: the average luminance of the grating; the luminance profile of the gratings, usually sine or square waves; the blur level of the optical system; the transparency of the optical media (Kolb et al., 2007).

Directly related to the transmission of light through the different structures of the eye, CSF is reduced in any of the processes that affect their transparency (corneal nebulae and leukomas, cataracts, opacification of the vitreous body) or prevent stimuli from reaching the retina (e.g. absence or ectopia of the pupil), as well as due to imperfections in the formation of images by the optical system of the eye (ametropia and aberrations). It is basically dependent on the functioning of the retina and visual pathways, and is also reduced when these structures are affected (detachments, degeneration, inflammation and scarring of the central part of the retina, optic neuritis or impairment of axons related to ganglion cells in the fovea, lesions affecting the visual cortex or other parts, etc.), or when neural development is imperfect (e.g. amblyopia) (Bicas, 2002).

At low luminance levels, the maximum contrast sensitivity is approximately 8 percent and the maximum resolution is approximately 6 cpg (figure 10). At higher luminance levels, CS increases at all spatial frequencies, the FSC peak reaches only 0.5% contrast (Kolb et al., 2007) and the highest spatial frequency reaches between 50 and 60 cycles per degree, which corresponds to the highest spatial resolution capacity under these conditions (Kolb et al., 2007; Schwartz, 2004).

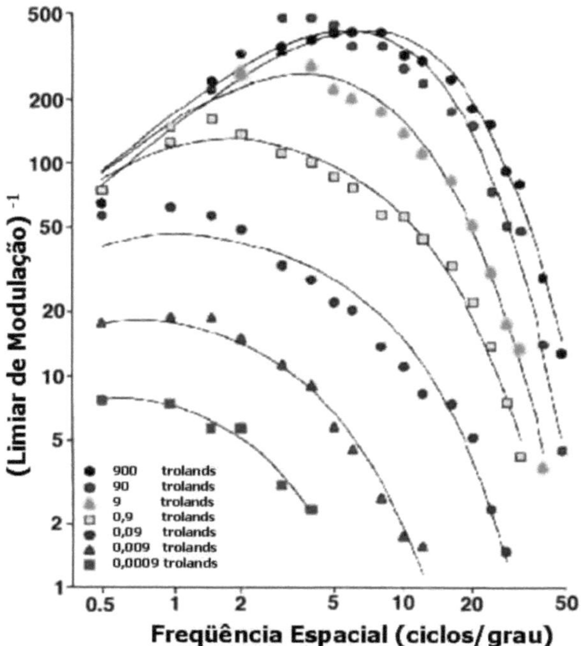

Fig. 10 - FSC showing the change in format to low-pass at low luminances and band-pass at high luminances.

(Kolb et al., 2007**webvision.med.utah.edu/KallSpatial.html**

Humans detect a grid of 4 cycles per degree at lower contrast levels than those required for the detection of other spatial frequencies, i.e. the peak of CS occurs at approximately 4 cpg (Schwartz, 2004).

As previously reported, the AV measure corresponds to the visual system's highest resolution capacity, and as it is generally obtained using optotypes with high levels of contrast with the background, it corresponds to the FSC cut-off at high spatial frequencies, using optotypes instead of gratings (Schwartz, 2004). AV therefore corresponds to just one point on the FSC (Figure 11).

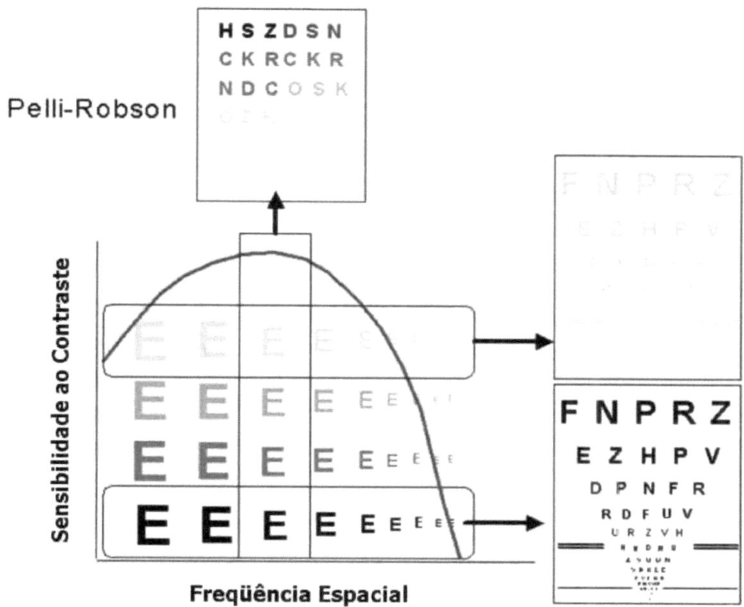

Fig. 11 - High and low contrast AV tables (right), and Pelli-Robson SC table (above), represented in a single AV and SC table (center) (Liu, C., 2007).

http://www.bsrs2000.fsnet.co.uk/new page 13.htm

By measuring the complete CSF, it is possible to differentiate between situations in which there are losses in the middle or low spatial frequencies and not in the high ones, or the opposite. This may be due to the fact that there are different groups of neurons for processing different spatial frequencies, according to the Multiple Channel Theory (Campbell, 1974; Cornsweet, 1970). This theory, created by (Campbell & Robson, 1968), is based on experiments in which CBF measured in subjects adapted to a certain spatial frequency showed a decrease in the region of the adapted spatial frequency, compared to CBF measured without this adaptation.

Based on these results, Campbell & Robson (1968) hypothesized that there are a number of separate channels in the visual system, each of which is tuned to a small group of spatial frequencies. Thus, some channels are specific to low frequencies, others to medium frequencies, and others to high frequencies. The complete sensitivity curve is given by the sensitivity peaks of each of the channels (figure 12).

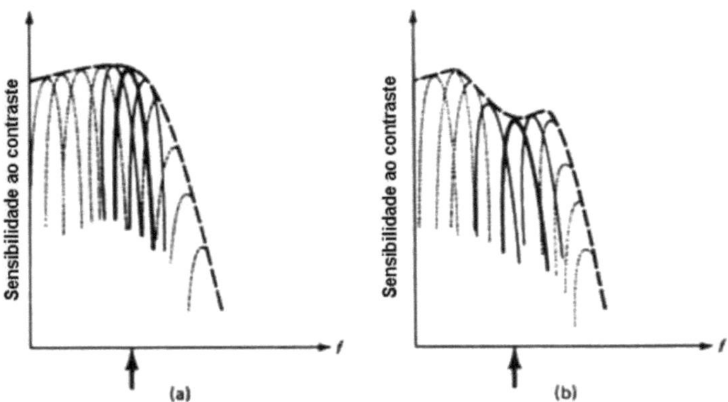

Fig. 12 - (a) The FSC is made up of several channels selective for spatial frequencies following the Multiple Channel Theory. (b) After adapting a specific spatial frequency, the FSC is lowered only in the region where this spatial frequency is located (Campbell et al., 1968).

The Multiple Channel Theory is reinforced by studies that report different critical periods of development in the same visual function and between different visual functions. Harwerth et al. (1986) found, after different periods of monocular deprivation in *Macaca mulatta*, different critical developmental periods for the following visual functions: scotopic spectral sensitivity (up to 3 months), photopic spectral sensitivity (up to 6 months), spatial vision (up to 25 months), binocularity (over 25 months). In addition, losses in spatial vision were greater at medium and high spatial frequencies than at lower frequencies. Losses increased with the length of the deprivation period in all the visual functions assessed.

I . 3 - The Contrast Sensitivity Function in Different Pathologies

Among the important aspects that can be assessed using CSF, it is worth highlighting the damage to visual perception caused by degenerative diseases, heavy metal poisoning, diabetes, the processes of demyelination of the visual pathways and also cortical lesions, which are common in human clinical practice (Rodrigues et al., 2007; Santos & Simas, 2001; Ventura et al., 2005). Examples of some alterations in the CS due to pathologies can be seen in figure 13. Patients with multiple sclerosis have discrete losses in the low spatial frequencies in CS (figure 13 -B), while patients with cataracts show a reduction in CS in all spatial frequencies (figure 1 3-C). Mild refractive error or amblyopia leads to a CSF similar to curve "D" in figure 13, with a loss in the high spatial frequencies. With greater refractive errors or severe amblyopia, the resulting CSF is similar to curve "C" in figure 13, i.e. loss at all spatial frequencies (Kolb et al., 2007).

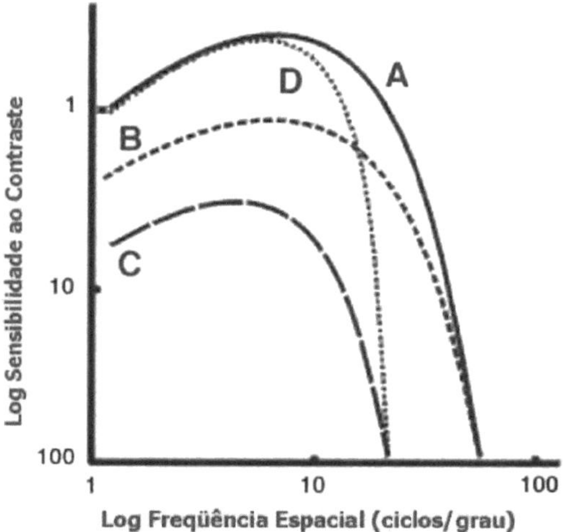

Fig. 13 - Examples of how the CSF (A) is altered due to diseases such as multiple sclerosis (B), cataracts (C), and refractive error or amblyopia (D).

(Kolb et al., 2007**webvision.med.utah.edu/KallSpatial.html**

Patients with cataracts in the early stages do not show CS losses at low frequencies, but as the disease progresses, losses occur at all spatial frequencies (Elliott & Situ, 1998).

Patients with meridional amblyopia show obvious abnormalities in the detection of contrast thresholds (StJohn, 1997).

Carriers of the mitochondrial DNA mutation that causes Leber's Hereditary Optic Neuropathy (NOHL), with normal AV, show losses in chromatic and luminance CS in all spatial frequencies evaluated by (Ventura et al., 2005).

CS measurement has also proved to be an important tool in detecting and monitoring visual dysfunction in patients with pituitary adenoma. Porciatti et al. (1999) evaluated the CS of patients with this diagnosis using two types of visual stimuli: a large (0.3 cpg), dynamic sinusoidal grid (with a temporal modulation of 10 Hz), defined as a Magnocellular stimulus; and a thinner (2.0 cpg), static one, defined as a Parvocellular stimulus. The results indicated that pituitary adenoma can cause significant dysfunction in the visual pathways in many patients without chiasmatic compression, and with normal acuity and visual field.

Acquired conditions such as chemical intoxication have been described in the literature as interfering with CSF. Lamp factory workers diagnosed with chronic mercurialism were evaluated for CS using psychophysical and electrophysiological methods and both showed a reduction in this visual function

(Ventura et al., 2005).

I . 4 - The Function of Contrast Sensitivity in Visual Development

In addition to its usefulness in assessing different pathologies, FSC can be used to study the development of the human visual system, or visual perception of shapes in infants (Adams & Courage, 2002; Allen, Tyler, & Norcia, 1996; Banks & Salapatek, 1976; Jackson et al, 2003; Kelly, Borchert, & Teller, 1997; Kelly & Chang, 2000; Montés-Micó & Ferrer-Blasco, 2001; Norcia, Tyler and Hamer, 1990; Oliveira et al, 2004; Rasengane, Allen, & Manny, 1997; Shannon, Skoczenski, & Banks, 1996) because many aspects responsible for the emergence of visual perception, such as the electrical responses of the retina, AV, stereopsis, color vision, temporal resolution, visual field, and CS itself, as previously pointed out, are all reduced in childhood compared to adult performance (Allen, Banks, & Norcia, 1993; Allen, Tyler, & Norcia, 1996; Atkinson and Braddick, 1989; Banks and Salapatek, 1976; Berezovsky et al., 1995; Berezovsky et al, 2003; Dobson & Teller, 1978; Hamer et al, 1989; Harvey et al, 1997; Jongmans et al, 1996; Kelly, Borchert, & Teller, 1997; Kos-Pietro et al, 1997; Morante et al, 1982; Moskowitz & Sokol, 1980; Norcia & Tyler, 1985; Rasengane, Allen, & Manny, 1997; Santos & Simas, 2001; Shannon, Skoczenski, & Banks, 1996; Teller, 1990; Teller, 1998).

The assessment of visual development in humans is extremely important for the following reasons: Firstly, if there is a critical period in which Vulnerability to a possible interruption of normal visual development is highest, it must coincide with a period of active visual development. Secondly, the basis of treatment for visual disorders depends critically on knowledge of normal developmental processes (Bradley & Freeman, 1982).

I . 5 - Human Visual Development

The visual processing hierarchy most commonly used in studies of the visual development of newborns and children is characterized by a division into three stages: early, middle and late. The progression from early to late stage corresponds to the complexity of the information extracted at each level. Vision, from the earliest stage, begins in the retina and continues through the lateral geniculate nucleus and the primary visual cortex. At this stage, attributes of visual stimuli such as orientation, direction of movement and disparity are extracted from retinal images. At the middle level, processing extends to the first two layers of the extra-striate visual areas, with information on shape, contour, the relationship between the figure and the background, symmetry between objects, and surface depth, but without including the identity of the objects in the scene. Object identification (object recognition), which involves not only visual perception but also memory, occurs in conjunction with higher visual associative areas and corresponds to the late stage of visual processing (Norcia & Manny, 2003).

The immaturity of the optical media of the eye, the mechanisms of accommodation, as well as refractive errors due to astigmatism, which are very common in children, associated with neural factors such as the immaturity of the retinal cones and their lower density in the fovea, the organization of the receptive fields of the ganglion cells of the human retina at birth, and the incomplete myelination of the axons of the optic nerve fibres potentially limit visual information even before it reaches the lateral geniculate nucleus and the superior colliculus, and subsequently the primary visual cortical area, which are also immature at birth (Atkinson & Braddick, 1989). Braddick, 1989).

Maurer et al. (1999), in a high-impact study published in the journal Science, showed that the post-natal development of vision depends on stimulation with spatio-temporal patterns present in the normal visual situation. They compared the VA of newborns diagnosed with cataracts in one or both eyes before and after surgical removal of the cataract, which deprived them of this stimulation. VA was measured immediately after the fitting of an appropriate contact lens, a few days after surgery. In this first assessment, the children's VA was compared to that of children who had a normal post-natal visual experience. The VA of the operated children was close to that of the newborn, regardless of their age, which varied between 1 and 9 months. The authors therefore showed that in the absence of visual stimuli, the VA of humans does not show any postnatal improvement. One hour after inserting the lens, the children were assessed again and the results showed that AV had already improved by approximately 0.4 octaves. The result proves that the nervous system reacts immediately to the presentation of such stimuli, and is able to promote rapid AV development.

The hypothesis that changes occur in the brain as a result of visual experience emerged around 1815 with Spurzheim (Diamond, 2001). Today it is known that while the encephalon has a relatively constant macro-structural organization, the cerebral cortex, with its complex micro-architecture and unknown potential, is strongly shaped by experiences even before birth, during youth, and indeed throughout life (Diamond, 2001).

The limited behavioral repertoire of newborns and the difficulty of assessing them have led visual scientists to develop adaptations of classic psychophysical and electrophysiological tests for newborns and pre-verbal children. The different methods - electrophysiological or behavioral - used to access visual functions evidently correspond to different stages in the hierarchy of visual processing (Norcia & Manny, 2003).

The first visual measurements of children were carried out in the 1950s with the Forced Choice Preferential Gaze technique (Fantz, 1958 apud Teller, 1997). In this technique, infants are confronted with a series of pairs of standardized stimuli while adults observe various aspects of their ocular behavior (direction of the first gaze, gaze time for each stimulus, and the number of times the infants look at each stimulus). This technique has been adapted for children over 5 months old who do not cooperate with all the stages of the test of their own free will. The adaptation includes the use of operant reinforcement after the trials, and the test is now called Operant Preferential Gaze (Mayer & Dobson, 1982). The length of time required to apply the Forced Choice Preferential Gaze and Operant Preferential Gaze techniques was very significant.

The Preferential Operant test led researchers to develop another methodological adaptation for the test, and the Teller acuity cards were created (McDonald et al., 1985) with the aim of adapting the test to pediatric ophthalmology clinical practice. In this adaptation, a set of cards with grids of different spatial frequencies was presented to the child, and with each hit (observation of the stimulus) finer grids (with a higher spatial frequency) were presented until their sensitivity threshold was reached, and the spatial frequency of the last card correctly observed by the child corresponded to an estimate of their acuity (figure 14).

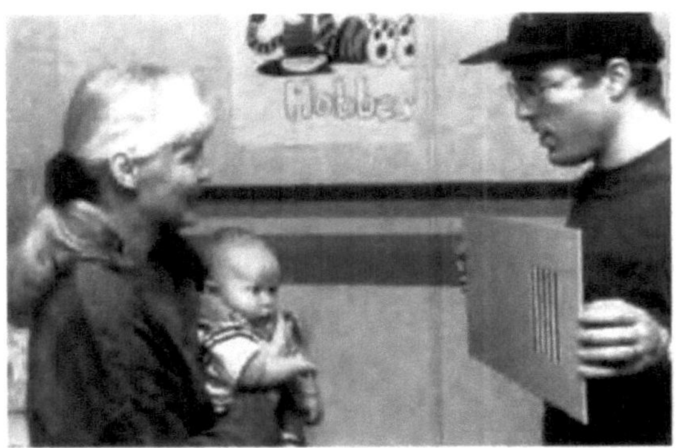

Fig. 14 - AV test with Teller's acuity cards (Teller, 1997).

Results from a series of validations of Teller's acuity cards have shown that acuities can be estimated in less than 5 minutes and intra-observer and inter-observer variability is very low (e.g. Salomao & Ventura, 1995; Mayer et al., 1995).

Subsequently, two other techniques were developed to assess vision in children: Optokinetic Nystagmus, performed through reflex eye movements related to stimuli presented in motion, and Visual Cortical Potential (VCP), performed through electrodes that capture cortical electrical activity related to standardized stimuli.

Preferential gaze and PVCP are related to the initial stage of the visual processing hierarchy, while optokinetic nystagmus is difficult to classify within this hierarchy due to the possible involvement of subcortical mechanisms used to control eye movements (Norcia & Manny, 2003).

Dobson & Teller (1978) carried out a review with the aim of comparing the development of VA during the first semester of life as measured by the Preferential Gaze, Optokinetic Nystagmus and PVCP techniques, and concluded that there is agreement between these measures. However, despite the agreement, there were differences in the values found in each test. The Preferential Gaze and Optokinetic Nystagmus results were very similar, but the PVCP results showed a tendency to rise. The differences in PVCP results can be attributed to factors such as:

- the nature of the visual stimulus presented, commonly stationary gratings in behavioral methods and temporally modulated gratings in electrophysiological methods;
- the use of average values for the electrophysiological recording signal, in addition to the summation of signals over the entire visual field;
- electrophysiological methods, such as PVCP, reflect only the sensory aspects of the visual system, from the photoreceptors to the occipital cortex, while behavioral methods, such as Preferential Gaze, possibly involve other structures such as the associative and motor cortex;
- the level of the response criterion chosen by each researcher in each method also shows significant differences (Dobson & Teller, 1978; Sokol, 1978; Teller, 1997).

The VA of a newborn has a limitation of approximately 50 times when compared to the same visual function of an adult, but this function shows rapid development in the first six months of life (Dobson & Teller, 1978; Maurer et al., 1999; Norcia & Tyler, 1985; Salomao & Ventura, 1995; Schwartz, 2004; Sokol, 1978).

Salomao & Ventura (1995) developed standards for the Teller acuity cards. They evaluated the VA of children divided into age groups every 2 months and showed that there is a significant difference in the VA of 2-month-olds compared to 4-month-olds, and 4-month-olds compared to 6-month-olds, but above 6 months the gradual increase in VA was not significant, confirming the important increase in this visual function in the first semester of life (figure 15).

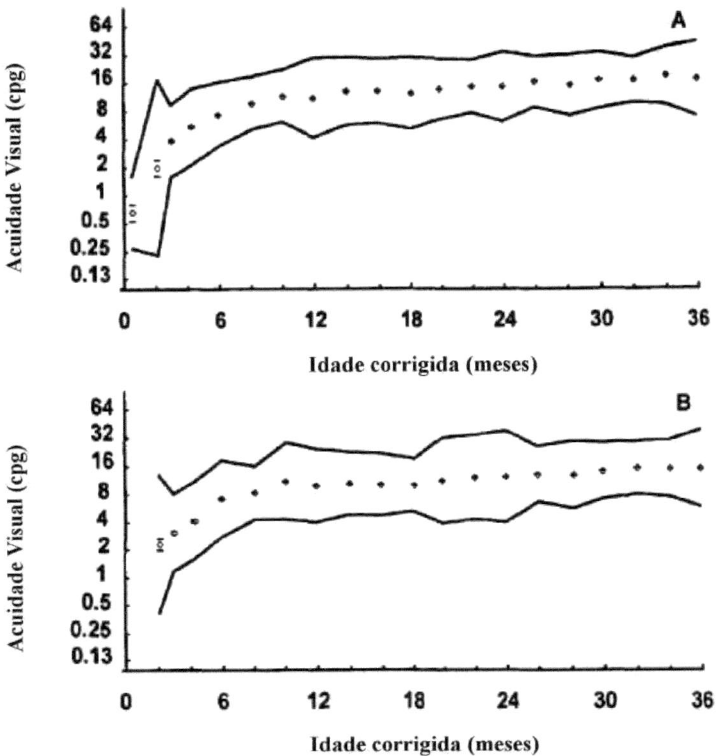

Fig. 15 - A. Mean binocular acuity ± SD and tolerance limits for 90% of the population with 95% probability, based on data from 646 healthy babies and children, as a function of age. B. Mean monocular acuity ± SP and tolerance limits for 90% of the B. Mean monocular acuity ± EP and tolerance limits for 90% of the population with 95% probability, based on data from 624 healthy babies and children, as a function of age. (Salomao and Ventura, 1995)

There is a prolonged period of post-natal development, extending from the third to the fifth year of life, in which spatial vision reaches adult levels (Boothe et al., 1988). The VA of a healthy adult is equal to or greater than 30 cpg (equivalent to 20/20 on the Snellen scale) while a healthy child during the first month of life resolves approximately 1 cpg (20/600 Snellen) reaching adult values around the third full year, in behavioral measures (Teller, 1990).[1]

Standards for Teller's acuity cards were also carried out by Mayer et al. (1995) as shown in figure 16, and their results exemplify the findings of Boothe et al. (1988), Teller (1990) and Salomao and

1 AV thresholds expressed in visual angle are converted to Snellen acuity by multiplying the minutes of arc by a factor of 20. This produces the denominator of the Snellen fraction. A Snellen acuity of 20/20 is equivalent to a visual resolution threshold of 1 arc minute (Sokol, 1978).

Ventura (1995).

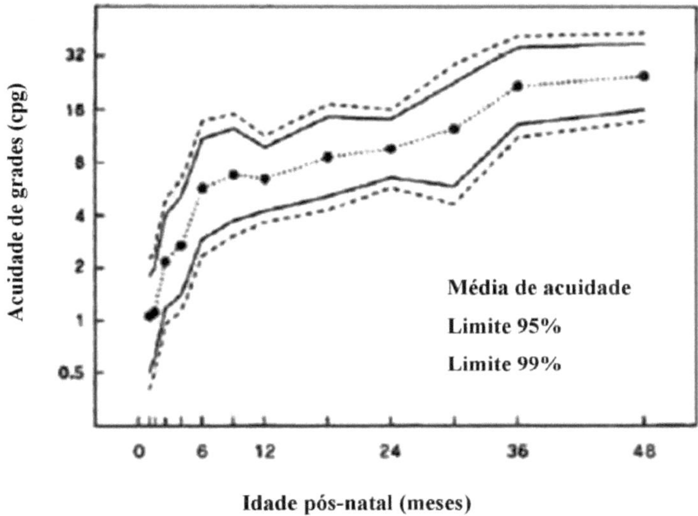

Fig. 16 - Norms for the AV Test with Teller's acuity cards, carried out by Mayer et al., (1995) (Teller, 1997).

Similar to the VA, the CBF, which is considerably immature at birth in terms of both shape and sensitivity, also develops rapidly in the first year of life (Norcia, Tyler & Hamer, 1990; Oliveira et al., 2004). The first measurements of the CSF in children were made approximately three decades ago by (Atkinson, Braddick, & Braddick, 1974; Banks & Salapatek, 1976), who assessed children at 2 months of age and found the CSF to be considerably reduced compared to that of adults (figure 17).

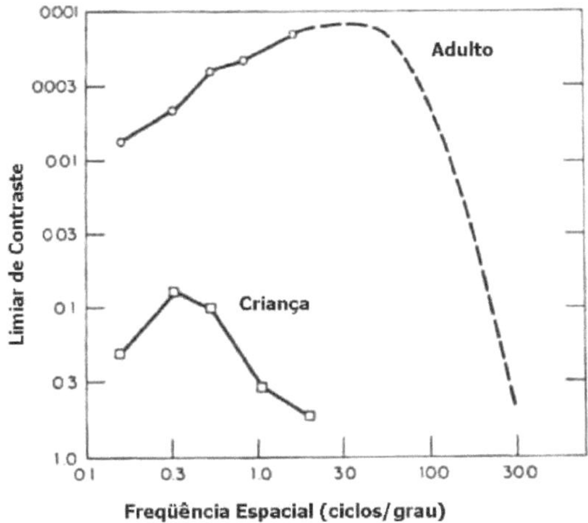

Fig. 17- Average CBF for 2-month-olds and adults. Contrast magnitudes are plotted against spatial frequencies. The dotted line represents a typical portion of the CBF at high spatial frequencies in adults (Banks & Salapatek 1976).

In 1977, Atkinson, Braddick, & Moar showed that there is a qualitative and quantitative development in the CSF during the first weeks of life by evaluating children at 5, 8 and 12 weeks of age and associated this improvement in the CSF of children in the second month of life with the rapid and comprehensive development that occurs in the vision-related regions of the human nervous system during this period.

Studies on the development of the CBF have also been carried out in animal models. Boothe et al. (1988) evaluated three parameters of the CBF: the value of the peak sensitivity, the spatial frequency at which the peak sensitivity is found, and the spatial frequencies of the *Macaca nemestrina* pass band. The authors found a rapid development between the tenth and twentieth week of life, followed by a gradual, slower development after this period. The three FSC parameters evaluated showed a similar development pattern (figure 18).

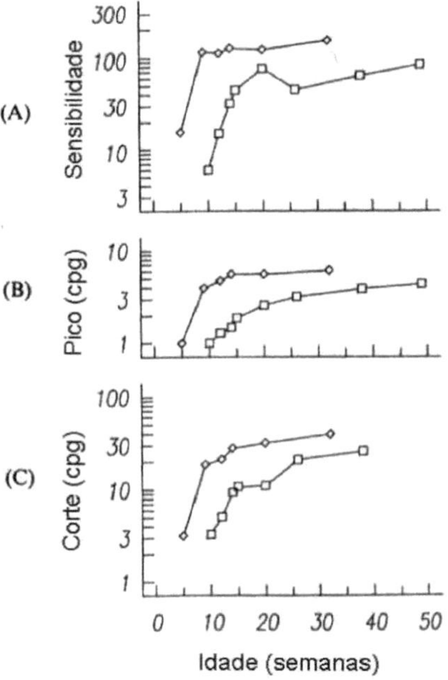

Fig. 18- Development of three parameters of the FSC *of Macaca nemestrina*: the value of the peak sensitivity (A), the spatial frequency at which the peak sensitivity is found (B), and the spatial frequencies of the passband (C). The data plotted are from two representative monkeys: the fastest developing (◊), and the slowest developing (□) (Boothe et al., 1988).

Montés-Micó & Ferrer-Blasco (2001), using the *Vistech Contrast Sensitivity Test System*, assessed children between 3 and 7 years of age monocularly and found a discreet and slow development in CSF during this period.

Using a test developed by the authors themselves to assess FSC based on Teller's visual acuity cards, Adams & Courage (2002) assessed children aged 4 to 9 and adults. They then added these data to those of two previous studies (Adams et al., 1992; Adams & Courage, 1993) in which they assessed babies aged between 1 month and 3 years. The results showed a qualitative and quantitative development of the CSF in this period, with emphasis on the complete maturation of this function occurring at 9 years of age and the increase in CS for the highest spatial frequencies at the highest ages (figure 19).

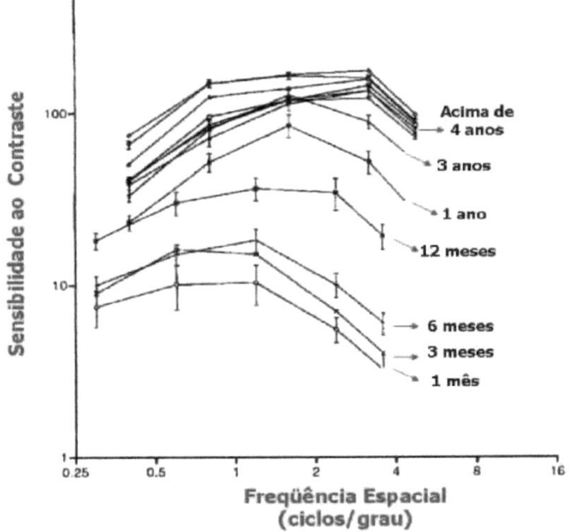

Fig. 19- FSC development from the first month of life to maturity with the averages and standard errors of each spatial frequency at each age assessed (Adams & Courage, 2002).

Temporal resolution measurements were carried out on children to check their critical fusion frequency of intermittent stimuli (temporal variation). The results showed a good resolution in the first month of life, of approximately 40 Hz, evolving to approximately 50 Hz at 2 months and 52 Hz in the third month, approaching that of adults who reach 55 Hz (Regal, 1981).

Measurements of temporal contrast sensitivity or temporal FSC provide a more complete description of temporal vision than just the measurement of critical fusion frequency at maximum contrast. They were assessed for development in children aged between 2 and 4 months, using a variant of the Preferential Gaze technique. The results showed that this function, like spatial FSC, changes as age increases (Rasengane, Allen & Manny, 1997).

Three-month-old children and adults were assessed for temporal CSF with chromatic and luminance stimuli that included moving gratings and counter-phase gratings, and the results, shown in figure 20, show a decrease in the children's sensitivity to both stimuli and both types of gratings, but no change in the peak frequency of sensitivity, as occurs with the development of spatial CSF (Dobkins & Teller, 1995; Dobkins, Lia & Teller, 1997).

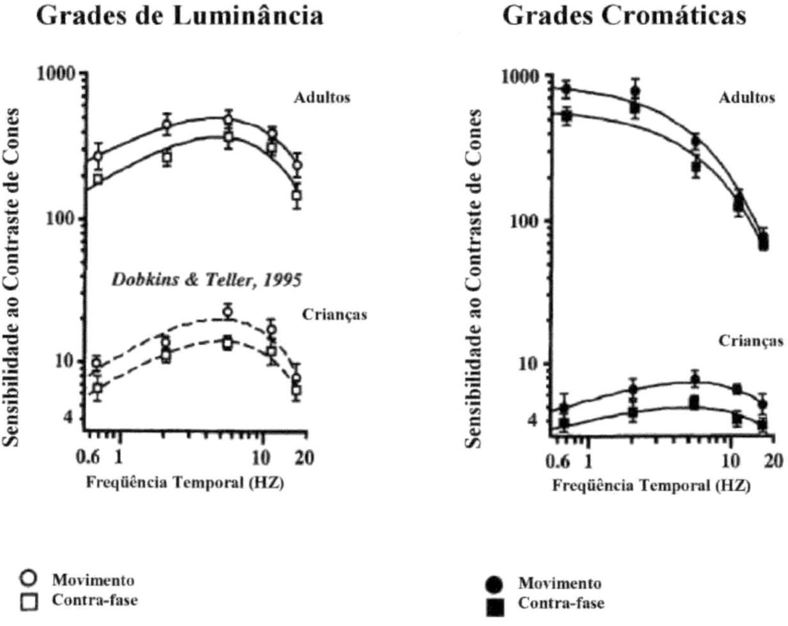

Fig. 20 - Chromatic and luminance temporal FSC with moving and counterphase grating stimuli, measured by Dobkins, Lia & Teller (1995) and Dobkins & Teller (1997) (Teller, 1997).

As can be seen in the work of Dobkins & Teller (1997), children as young as three months show sensitivity to chromatic stimuli. There is a great deal of scientific agreement between laboratories and different techniques, suggesting that green-red discrimination emerges in the second month of life in most children. The emergence of discrimination on the tritan axis is less studied, and the few existing studies present many contradictions (Teller, 1997).

Stereopsis, the ability to perceive depth based on binocular disparity, has also been the subject of research into visual development. Many researchers have shown, using different techniques, the absence of stereopsis responses in almost all children under 3 months of age, and the beginning of this ability between the third and fifth month of life, but with an abrupt developmental course in relation to the development of grating visual acuity, reaching adult values by the sixth month of life (Norcia & Manny, 2003; Teller 1997).

Like stereopsis, vernier acuity - a measure of the smallest visible separation between two stimuli - has a more abrupt developmental course than grating acuity, but less abrupt than that found for stereopsis. Vernier acuity reaches adult levels around 60 months of age, in a similar way to grating acuity (Teller 1997).

The development of visual functions in premature infants presents conflicting results in the literature. While some authors find impairment, others find little or no loss.

Jongmans et al. (1996) found a decrease (classified as medium level in most cases) in VA, as well as altered stereopsis in 6-year-old children born prematurely, but several important factors such as refractive error, strabismus, amblyopia, and damage to the post-chiasmatic region of the visual pathway may have contributed to these children's altered results.

Salomao et al. (2001) evaluated preterm patients with poor visual attention and/or lack of fixation and retrochiasmatic lesion, but with normal fundus, and found bilateral vision loss and/or amblyopia, corroborating the diagnosis of visual cortical lesion in this group of patients.

Visual evaluations in prematurely born children with visual cortical lesions without primary ocular pathologies were also carried out by Pike et al. (1994), who found visual losses associated to a greater degree with ischemic cortical lesions than with hemorrhagic lesions.

Morante et al. (1982) evaluated visual acuity and pattern preference functions in term and premature newborns. The premature infants were classified into two groups: a low-risk group (with normal neurological examination findings), and a group with abnormal neurological examination findings (higher-risk group). Preterm infants in the low-risk group differed from controls only in the assessment by pattern preference, as they did not show differences in VA measurements. Preterm infants in the group with abnormal neurological examinations, on the other hand, showed lower results than controls both in the assessment by pattern preference and in the VA assessment.

Mash & Dobson (1998) evaluated the VA of 129 children born prematurely and/or who had suffered some kind of perinatal complication, because these children are more prone to ocular and visual alterations, and found a small number of subjects with altered VA.

Van Hof-van Duin & Mohn (1986) demonstrated that VA assessed by the forced-choice preferential gaze technique shows similar results for premature babies with minimal perinatal complications and babies born at term.

The responses of rods, maximal responses, and cones with 30 Hz *flicker* in the full-field electroretinogram, mass electrical signals generated by the retina in response to visual stimuli, showed similar waveforms and parameters between healthy premature newborns at 5 weeks corrected age and controls of the same age (Berezovsky et al., 2003).

The latencies of the reverse pattern PVCP responses showed no significant differences between premature and term infants of the same gestational age (Kos-Pietro et al., 1997). No acceleration in the development of visual resolution or early decrease in response latency as a result of premature infants' early visual experience was also observed in this group of patients (Kos-Pietro et al., 1997).

Rudduck & Harding (1994), also using reverse pattern PVCP to assess premature babies over 30 weeks gestational age and term babies, found similar PVCP morphology in the two groups, although the premature babies showed an increase in amplitude and a reduction in response latency as gestational age increased.

Amplitude and latency of the N1 and P1 components of reverse pattern PVCP responses to specific stimuli to assess the magnocellular and parvocellular pathways were evaluated by Hammarrenger et al. (2007) in healthy term and premature infants also born with very low birth weight. The age group of premature infants over 16 weeks of corrected age showed lower results than term infants for stimuli associated with the magnocellular pathway.

Premature infants were also assessed for CBF in a computerized psychophysical test, but the tests were carried out between 7 and 13 years of age and not during the developmental phase of the function. The results showed a slight improvement in CBF with increasing age, and the CBF of premature infants showed no statistically significant differences when compared to that of full-term subjects (Jackson et al., 2003).

Another study with premature infants and children born small for their gestational age was carried out during the subjects' adolescence and assessed visual functions such as VA, FSC using the *Vistech* test cards, visual field, refractive errors and the use of visual correction. Lower results were found in the VA, FSC and use of visual correction of the premature infants compared to the control group. The group born small for gestational age had a higher risk of hyperopia than the control group (Lindqvist et al., 2007).

Given all these factors that can affect children born prematurely, the use of equipment that provides more complete functional diagnoses than those normally obtained in clinical practice is of great value. Table 1 below summarizes the data from the studies described.

Table 1 - Summary of data from studies on babies born prematurely			
Authors	**Sample**	**Measured function**	**Result ***
Jongmans et al.,	Premature babies	AV, Stereopsis	Decreased

1996			Decreased
Salomao et al., 2001	Premature infants with cortical damage	AV	Decreased
Pike et al., 1994	Premature infants with cortical damage	AV	Decreased
Morante et al., 1982	Low and high risk premature babies	AV Pattern preference	Decreased
Mash & Dobson, 1998	Premature babies	AV	Little change
Van Hof-van Duin & Mohn, 1986	Premature babies	AV	No change
Berezovsky et al., 2003	Healthy premature babies	ERG	No change
Kos-Pietro et al., 1997	Healthy premature babies	Reverse pattern PVCP	No change
Rudduck & Harding, 1994	Premature babies over 30 weeks old	Reverse pattern PVCP	No change in wave morphology
Hammarrenger et al., 2007	Very low birth weight premature babies assessed at 16 weeks	Reverse pattern PVCP with stimuli for magno and parvo	Decreased stimulation of the magnocellular pathway
Jackson et al., 2003	Premature infants assessed from 7 to 13 years of age	FSC	No change
Lindqvist et al., 2007	Premature babies assessed in adolescence	VA, FSC, visual field, refractive error, visual correction	Decreased VA, FSC and use of vision correction, increased hyperopia

* compared to subjects born at term

I . 6 - Visual Cortical Potential (VCP)

The PVCP test allows for the diagnosis and monitoring of possible problems in the visual pathways. This test is non-invasive and relatively quick to perform, as well as not requiring much cooperation from the patient, as it is based on neural responses for which it is enough for the patient to look at the stimuli.

PVCP represents part of the activity of the visual cortex in response to visual information that passes through the optical media of the eye and is processed by the retina and the geniculo-striatal pathway (Norcia & Tyler, 1985). It is an electrophysiological signal recorded in the scalp using standardized electroencephalogram techniques (Harding et al., 1996). The presence of a provoked response indicates that the visual pathway has resolved the information from the stimulus to the point in the visual system where the response is generated (Norcia & Tyler, 1985).

Three types of stimulation are commonly used:

- PVCP by light pulses - diffuse light pulses of approximately 3 cd/m^2 with a maximum duration of 5 ms are presented by a xenon arc photostimulator and projected at least 20 degrees from the retina;
- PVCP by pattern reversal - black and white grids exceeding 15 degrees of visual angle are alternated temporally at a specified reversal rate (usually around 6 Hz) without modifying the average luminance of the screen, and the stimulus is defined in terms of the spatial frequency of these grids (the stimulus can also be a checkerboard pattern);
- PVCP by on/off pattern - a pattern (with stimuli similar to those of the reverse pattern) is presented for approximately 200 ms and then abruptly switched to an equiluminant diffuse background for about 400 ms without changing the average luminance of the screen (Harding et al., 1996).

In humans, PVCP has been used to assess the AV of grid resolution, especially in newborns and children. In contrast to the child's rapidly changing state and their fixation and attention, which are two parameters that are difficult to control, children have higher PVCP amplitudes than adults. This is partly due to the fact that the thickness of children's skull bones is less than that of adults. Thus the PVCP signals in children are even greater in relation to intrinsic brain noise (such as muscle activity) (Norcia et al., 1989).

Sokol (1978), using reverse pattern PVCPs on normal babies, observed that visual acuity improved from 20/150 at two months of age to a value of 20/20, equivalent to that of normal adults, around the sixth to eighth month of life, unlike behavioral methods which recorded VAs ranging from 20/600 to 20/400 at birth to 20/20 between 36 and 60 months of age (Birch & Bane, 1991; Courage & Adams, 1990).

The higher signal-to-noise ratio and the low fixation capacity of the stimuli by babies naturally led researchers to develop a computerized presentation methodology in which the parameters could automatically scan the range of interest and the resulting responses could at the same time be sent for real-time spectral analysis (online) (Norcia et al., 1989). This is what happens in a spatial frequency sweep PVCP scan. In this technique, grids (square wave or sine wave) are presented successively varying in spatial frequency, from low frequencies to high frequencies, in a range of frequencies around the AV, providing a measure of the sensory threshold. Alterations in these responses reflect damage or dysfunction of the visual pathways (Norcia et al., 1989). Instead of scanning across a range of spatial frequencies, the same can be done for a range of contrasts at a fixed spatial frequency, in an achromatic or chromatic situation. In this case, a contrast threshold is measured for each spatial frequency.

Scanning PVCPs have been used to evaluate functions such as AV (Allen, Tyler, & Norcia, 1996; da Costa et al., 2004; Hamer et al., 1989; Haro, 2003; Mazzitelli, 2002; Norcia & Tyler, 1985; Salomao et al, 2001; Shannon, Skoczenski & Banks, 1996), and luminance and/or chromaticity FSC (Allen, Tyler, & Norcia, 1996; Hamer et al., 1989; Haro, 2003; Kelly, Borchert, & Teller, 1997; Kelly & Chang, 2000; Norcia & Tyler, 1985; Norcia et al., 1989; Norcia, Tyler & Hamer, 1990; Oliveira et al., 2004).

Norcia & Tyler (1985) assessed the VA of 197 children between the first and 53th weeks of life using scanning PVCP, and found that around the eighth month of life, the first results showed VA values equivalent to those of an adult. Despite this, the average VA of the group aged between 8 and 13 months (approximately 20 cpg) did not reach the adult average (approximately 24 cpg) due to the low VA result (approximately 17 cpg) of the group of children aged around 12 months (n=11).

Hamer et al. (1989), using the same technique, found VA values equivalent to 14 cpg around the eighth month of life, unlike Norcia & Tyler (1985), who found 20 cpg, a value similar to that of adults, and the explanation for the difference in results lies in methodological differences. Norcia & Tyler (1985) used a VA growth curve based on the best estimated acuity result for each child, while Hamer et al. (1989) used the geometric mean of the estimated acuities. The authors also showed that there was no statistically significant difference between the results of monocular and binocular tests with the Scanning PVCP at any stage of visual development.

The development of grid-resolving AV was greater in the center than in the periphery of the visual field, while the development of SC was similar in the central and peripheral fields of vision, in children aged 10 to 39 weeks assessed with a variant of the Scanning PVCP (Allen, Tyler & Norcia, 1996).

Psychophysical and electrophysiological assessments (scanning PVCP) of the CSF in adults have been compared with each other and have shown that psychophysical sensitivity is slightly higher than electrophysiological sensitivity in this function (Norcia, Tyler & Hamer, 1990).

Comparisons between psychophysical and electrophysiological methods (scanning PVCP) were also carried out by Allen, Banks & Norcia (1993), who, unlike Norcia, Tyler & Hamer (1990), found no statistically significant differences between the results of the two methods for any of the achromatic and chromatic stimuli evaluated in adults.

Shannon, Skoczenski & Banks (1996) evaluated luminance CS at different spatial frequencies in 2- and 3-month-old infants and adults, using scanning PVCP and varying the luminance of the stimulus. As expected, they found that after an optimal luminance level, contrast thresholds decreased as luminance was increased, at all spatial frequencies, in both infants and adults. In conclusion, they reported that none of the models relating optical and receptor immaturities to spatial vision in children was able to explain the relationship between the retina's decreased ability to capture photons and CS.

Table 2 below summarizes the data from the studies carried out with PVCP.

Table 2 - Summary of data from studies carried out with Provoked Visual Cortical Potentials

Authors	**Sample**	**Measured function**	**Results**
Norcia & Tyler, 1985	Children between the first and 53rd week	AV	Development curve stabilizes in the 8th month of life at 20 cpg
Hamer et al., 1989	Children between 2 and 52 weeks	AV	Ditto with 14 cpg and greater AV development in the center than in the periphery
Allen, Banks & Norcia, 1993	Adults	AV	Results psychophysical shows higher CS than electrophysiological
Shannon, Skoczenski & Banks, 1996	Babies 2 and 3 months and adults	SC	After an ideal luminance level, the CS decreases with the increase in luminance
Allen, Banks & Norcia, 1993	Babies from 2 to 8 weeks	Chromatic SC	Lower than adult CS
Kelly, Borchert & Teller, 1997	Babies of 8, 14, 20 and 32 weeks and adults	SC chromatic and achromatic	Faster maturation of chromatic SC compared to achromatic SC
Norcia, Tyler and Hamer, 1990	Babies up to 30 weeks old	SC	Development of low frequencies up to the 10th° week and from high up to the 30th week
Kelly & Chang, 2000	Babies 14, 20 and 32	detection of chromatic	Contour detection does not

	weeks old	and luminance contours	differ according to age
Baraldi et al., 1981	Premature babies	AV measured by PCVP and Olhar Preferencial	AV best in Olhar Preferencial
Mirabella et al., 2006	Very low birth weight premature babies	AV, FSC, and vernier acuity	No change compared to terms
Haro, 2003	Premature babies with and without altered neuropsychomotor development	AV	Higher in rematuros without developmental change than in terms
Mazzitelli, 2002	Premature babies and terms	AV	AV does not differ between premature and term babies

Allen, Banks & Norcia (1993) showed that chromatic CS measured by scanning PVCP in children aged 2 to 8 weeks by varying the mixture of green and red components is lower than the sensitivity of adults.

Scanning PVCP was again used to assess the development of spatial, chromatic (green/red) and achromatic CSF in children aged 8, 14, 20 and 32 weeks and adults, revealing differences in both sensitivity and the shape of the sensitivity curve in achromatic and chromatic assessments in relation to age. In addition, the data suggested that the chromatic spatial CSF matured more quickly than the achromatic one, demonstrating the existence of distinct developmental stages for each visual function (Kelly, Borchert & Teller, 1997).

The detection of chromatic contours and luminance measured by scanning PVCP, unlike sensitivity thresholds, showed no significant changes in relation to age in children assessed at 14, 20 and 32 weeks (Kelly & Chang, 2000).

Another important study on the development of CSF using scanning PVCP was carried out by Norcia, Tyler & Hamer (1990), and showed that CS for lower spatial frequencies develops rapidly in the first 10 weeks after birth, unlike higher frequencies, which continue to develop until around 30 weeks of life, reaching the thresholds of a healthy adult. The results of this study were extremely higher than those obtained in the work by Pirchio et al. (1978), and these differences were attributed to the value of the

The luminance used by Norcia, Tyler & Hamer (1990) was 220 cd/m^2, approximately 50 times higher than that used by Pirchio et al. (1978). The FSC development time, which was faster in the study by Norcia, Tyler & Hamer (1990), also proved to be an important difference between these studies.

Scanning PVCP has also been used to assess visual development in babies born prematurely. Baraldi et al. (1981) compared full-term and premature infants using PVCP and forced-choice preferential gaze to measure VA, showing better VA in premature subjects assessed by the forced-choice preferential gaze method and no difference when assessed by PVCP.

VA, CSF and vernier acuity were assessed using the scanning PVCP method in healthy term and premature infants aged between 5 and 7 months and born with very low birth weight (< 1500g), and none of the three measurements showed a significant difference in thresholds when comparing the two groups of subjects. The authors only found differences in the amplitude of the responses, with premature infants showing better amplitudes in the contrast sensitivity and vernier acuity measurements, but without influencing the results of the measurements (Mirabella et al., 2006).

Haro (2003) traced the development of grid-resolving VA using the scanning PVCP method in babies born at term and prematurely with and without altered neuropsychomotor development. The results showed that AV at birth in preterm babies without neuropsychomotor developmental disorders is higher than in full-term babies, but the faster development of the full-term group corrects the difference in relation to these preterm babies. Preterm infants with altered neuropsychomotor development showed a decrease in VA from birth until the end of the first year of life when compared to the full-term group.

Another study on the development of grid-resolving AV by Mazzitelli (2002), which also used the scanning PVCP technique, showed that AV does not differ between children born at term and prematurely.

In conclusion, a number of studies have been carried out evaluating VA in almost all types of patients, including premature infants, but few studies have dealt with visual CSF, and far fewer have focused on premature infants.

The objective of evaluating CBF, in addition to VA, in premature infants is justified by the fact that no studies have been found measuring CBF in premature infants with the Scanning PVCP, and by the fact that the method of the Scanning PVCP provides a short time assessment of spatial vision in relation to VA and CS for non-verbal patients, minimizing the influences that can occur and interfere with the results of these same tests (VA and CS) by behavioral measures.

II - Objectives

The purpose of this study is to:

A - to determine the development of AV and CS functions at spatial frequencies of 0.2, 0.8, 2.0 and 4.0 cpg during the first year of life (with a greater focus on the ages of 4, 6 and 12 months) in preterm and full-term babies;

B - to determine whether or not there is a correlation between CBF values and the birth weight, Apgar score and gestational age of these premature infants.

III - Methods

III.1 - Participants

57 healthy babies of both sexes (31 males and 26 females), with no diagnosis of systemic or neurological diseases during their first year of life, were referred from the Pediatrics Department of the University Hospital of the University of Sao Paulo. The guardians of the babies who agreed to take part in the study signed an informed consent form and were made aware of all the procedures used.

The study was approved by the Ethics Committee of the University Hospital of USP (CEP 432/03).

The babies were previously separated into two groups: term babies (n=26) and premature babies (n=31). The babies were assessed for AV and CS functions at different ages, with a greater focus on 4, 6 and 12 months, and a total of 116 assessments were carried out, of which 49 were in term babies and 67 in premature babies. Prematurity was defined as birth at a gestational age of less than 37 weeks (7/7 days).

In addition to the babies, 23 healthy adults of both sexes took part in the experiments. AV was assessed in 9 (5 males and 4 females, mean age 21.9 years) of the 23 participants, and FSC in 14 (8 males and 6 females, mean age 39.5 years) at the same spatial frequencies tested in the infants.

The inclusion criteria were: ophthalmologic examination with normal fundus and available clinical and laboratory tests with no evidence of neurological or systemic diseases. All the premature babies underwent a skull ultrasound scan, and only those with normal results were selected for the study.

A female baby born prematurely had a low VA for her age in her second test session and her two tests (VA and CS), carried out in a previous session and in the session in which she had a low VA, were excluded from the data analysis.

Four babies, 2 born at term and 2 born prematurely, were brought in for their first examination at over 12 months of age, and their AV and SC tests were not selected for the work.

During 13 CS tests, the babies were unable to complete the test in all 4 spatial frequencies with the appropriate criteria for data analysis, and the results of these spatial frequencies were excluded. The same occurred in 2 tests with full-term babies. This difference between the preterm and term tests is explained by the greater number of tests carried out on preterm babies before the age of 3 months, the age group in which most of the failures occurred in the evaluation of any of the 4 spatial frequencies (7 of the 13 failures in preterm babies). In the period before 3 months, 18 tests were carried out on premature babies and only 12 on full-term babies.

Table 3 shows the demographic data of all the full-term babies assessed during the study.

Table 3 - Demographic data of babies born at term							
Code	Sex	Class	Date	Date	Age	Apgar	Weight
			Birth	Likely	Gestational	1 /5 / 10	(grs)
1	F	T	18/02/2001	18/02/2001	40	7 8	2280
2	F	T	17/04/2001	17/04/2001	40	8 10	2885
3	M	T	03/07/2001	07/07/2001	39	9 10	3230
4	M	T	13/12/2001	16/12/2001	39	8 9	3700
5	F	T	21/06/2002	27/06/2002	40	7 9	3890
6	M	T	10/12/2002	10/12/2002	40	9 10	3170
7	M	T	20/12/2002	10/01/2003	37	9 10	2865
8	F	T	18/02/2003	25/02/2003	39	9 10	3550
9	F	T	27/03/2003	10/04/2003	38	8 10	3330
10	M	T	22/05/2003	22/05/2003	40	8 9	3750
11	M	T	06/06/2003	08/06/2003	39	8 9	3145
12	M	T	09/10/2003	12/10/2003	40	4 6	3025
13	F	T	06/04/2004	07/04/2004	39	7 9	2745
14	F	T	05/06/2004	05/06/2004	40	4 7	3420
15	M	T	11/08/2004	18/08/2004	39	8 9	3480
16	M	T	05/09/2004	18/09/2004	38	7 9	2580
17	M	T	13/09/2004	15/09/2004	39	8 9	2495
18	F	T	29/12/2004	12/01/2005	38	9 10	2940
19	M	T	10/04/2005	17/04/2005	39	8 9	3560
20	F	T	25/04/2005	25/04/2005	40	9 10	3160
21	F	T	06/05/2005	06/05/2005	40	8 9	3255
22	M	T	19/06/2005	03/07/2005	38	9 10	3260
23	M	T	23/10/2005	30/10/2005	39	10 10	3200
24	M	T	31/10/2005	07/11/2005	39	10 10	3440
25	F	T	14/11/2005	21/11/2005	39	10 10	2975
26	M	T	20/11/2005	20/11/2005	40	9 10	3150

Table 4 shows the demographic data of all the premature babies assessed during the study.

Table 4 - Demographic data of babies born prematurely							
Code	Sex	Class	Date	Date	Age	Apgar	Weight
			Birth	Likely	Gestational	1 /5 / 10	(grs)
27	M	P	04/05/2001	10/08/2001	27	5 7	1215
28	M	P	16/05/2001	30/06/2001	32	6 9	1315
29	M	P	30/07/2001	07/09/2001	35	9 10	1720
30	F	P	14/08/2001	22/09/2001	34	6 8	970
31	M	P	02/10/2001	04/11/2001	35	8 9	1490
32	M	P	23/11/2001	18/12/2001	36	5 8	2135
33	M	P	27/11/2001	21/01/2002	33	7 9	2000
34	F	P	04/12/2001	15/01/2002	34	2 8	1770
35	F	P	19/12/2001	19/02/2002	32	6 8	1895
36	M	P	29/01/2002	30/03/2002	32	9 10	1025
37	F	P	10/03/2002	11/05/2002	31	6 7	1410
38	F	P	18/03/2002	17/04/2002	36	7 10	1885
39	F	P	03/04/2002	26/06/2002	29	6 8	990
40	M	P	27/08/2002	17/10/2002	32	7 9	1200
41	F	P	25/09/2002	20/12/2002	28	3 8	1100
42	M	P	25/10/2002	21/12/2002	32	8 9	1855
43	M	P	20/12/2002	27/02/2003	31	7 10	1650
44	F	P	20/12/2002	27/02/2003	31	7 9	1080
45	M	P	07/01/2003	15/03/2003	29	5 9	1415
46	M	P	16/02/2003	25/04/2003	30	3 5	960
47	F	P	17/03/2003	12/04/2003	36	8 10	2490
48	F	P	29/03/2003	08/05/2003	35	7 9	2360
49	M	P	12/04/2003	20/05/2003	35	9 9	1990
50	F	P	14/01/2004	09/04/2004	29	9 9	830

51	F	P	18/01/2004	16/02/2004	35	7	8	1620
52	F	P	09/05/2004	04/06/2004	36	7	7	1340
53	F	P	28/10/2004	21/12/2004	32	1	8	1130
54	M	P	28/10/2004	21/12/2004	32	4	9	1210
55	F	P	06/02/2005	06/04/2005	32	9	9	1880
56	M	P	15/12/2005	06/01/2006	36	7	9	2430
57	M	P	17/01/2006	08/02/2006	36	6	8	1210

* P - premature / T - term

III . 2 - Materials and Methods

III . 2 / A - Recording equipment and stimulus parameters

PVCPs measurements were obtained using 4 gold surface electrodes used for electroencephalography (Grass Gold Disc Electrodes - E6GH) placed on the scalp with an electrolytic cream and covered with cotton wool (Webril II). An elastic band (3M Coban SelfAdherent Wrap 158 1) was used to hold the electrodes in place. The active electrodes were placed at points O_1 and o_2, 2 - 3 cm to the right and left of the common reference electrode (o_z), which in turn was fixed 1 cm above the inion in the midline. A ground electrode was placed 2-3 cm above O_z following the standards suggested by ISCEV (*International Society for Clinical Electrophysiology of Vision)*, corresponding to the International 10/20 System (Odom et al., 2004). The placement of the electrodes and the test procedure can be seen in figures 21 A and B, and 22.

The electroencephalogram was amplified by a Neurodata Grass amplifier (12C-4-23 - gain = 10,000; attenuation of -3db at 1 and 100 Hz).

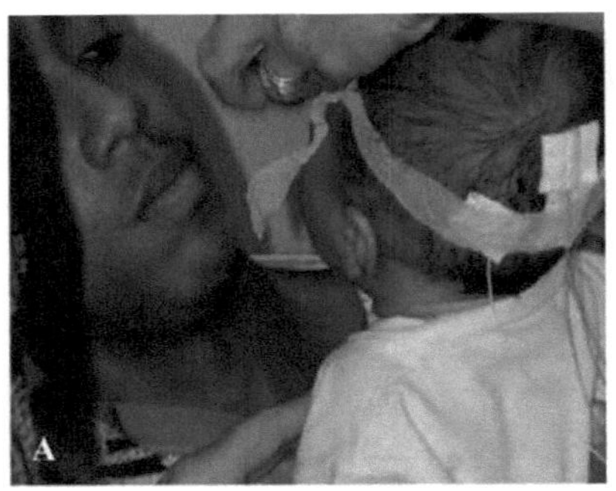

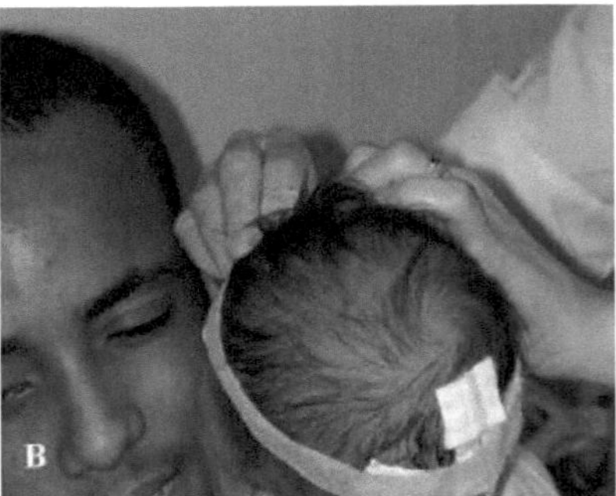

Fig. 21A and B - Cortical activity recording electrodes placed in the primary visual area to measure electrical responses to visual stimuli (Visual Evoked Potential) (Ventura, D. F., 2007).

http://www.ip.usp.br/laboratorios/visual/

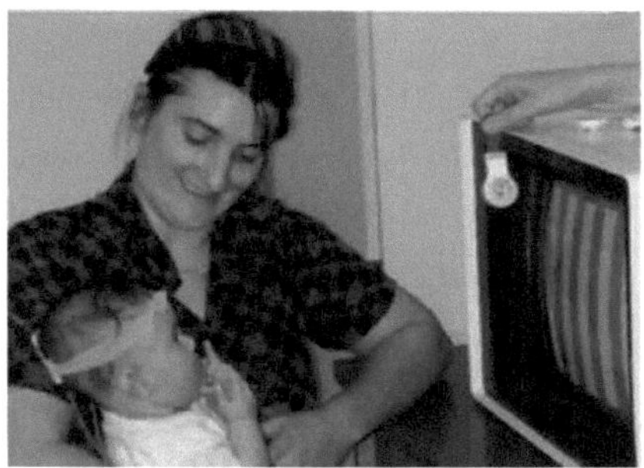

Fig. 22- The mother positions the child, trying to motivate them to look at the monitor where the stimuli are presented (Ventura, D. F., 2007).

http://www.ip.usp.br/laboratorios/visual/

The recording equipment also consists of a digitizer card for analyzing the acquired signals (see description in IV.2/C - Experimental Procedure) and a Power Macintosh model 7100/66 microcomputer. The system also includes a graphic interface for producing stimuli. This set is the NuDiva (Digital Infant Visual Assessment) version of the scanning PVCP system developed by Norcia & Tyler (1985).

III . *2 / B - Stimuli for Visual Acuity and Contrast Sensitivity*

The stimuli consisted of vertical square wave gratings for the VA assessment and vertical sinusoidal wave gratings for the CS assessment, presented on a high-resolution video monitor (Dotronix Model EM2400-D788), with an average luminance of 159.5 cd/m^2 comprising a visual angle of 33.6X25 degrees at 50 cm distance in the test for children and 16.8 X 12.5 degrees of visual angle at 100 cm distance for adults.

To assess AV, a spatial frequency sweep consisting of a sequence of ten spatial frequencies was presented at a rate of one frame per second, with ten reversal patterns in each spatial frequency. The temporal frequency of the reversals was 6 Hz. The contrast was kept fixed at 80%. The scanning range was selected with values that covered and exceeded the range of spatial frequency values that contained the AV threshold predicted for the age of the test subject based on preliminary laboratory standards (Haro, 2003), and its initial and final values could be set in the range of 0.2 to 40 cpg. For CS assessment, a contrast scan, consisting of a sequence of ten contrast levels, was presented at a rate of one frame per second, with ten reversal patterns in each contrast. The temporal frequency of the reversals was also 6 Hz. The spatial frequencies 0.2, 0.8, 2.0 and 4.0 cpg were evaluated. The scanning range used for each spatial frequency was selected, as in the AV measurement, with values that covered and exceeded the range of contrast values that the test subject could see, and their initial and final values could be set in the range of 100% to 0.7% contrast.

III . 2 / C - Experimental Procedure

In each session, the subjects' VA and CS were assessed. While the child was alert and carefully watching the video monitor, the experimenter activated the spatial frequency or contrast scan, depending on the test. The tests were carried out binocularly in a darkened room. The presentation of each stimulus for 1 second preceded the start of each scan of that stimulus.

At each stimulus presentation, small toys were shown in front of the video monitor and moved by the experimenter to attract the child's attention and keep them fixed close to the center of the screen.

III . 2 / D - Data analysis

The electroencephalogram was taken simultaneously from both channels and filtered in real time (sampling rate = 397 Hz) to isolate the PVCP. The electroencephalogram signal was digitized and analyzed using a discrete Fourier transform. The amplitude and phase of the Fourier components corresponding to the visual stimulation frequency (6Hz) and their harmonics were obtained. The analysis was carried out in a 1 Hz band window centered on the fundamental frequency (F1= 6Hz) and each harmonic (F2, F3, etc). For reverse stimulation patterns, the threshold is calculated based on F2 (12 Hz) since the symmetrical activation of the ON and OFF neural systems by the pattern produces symmetrical responses, causing a strong signal at this frequency (Norcia & Tyler, 1985; Hamer et al., 1989). On the other hand, ON-OFF stimulation produces a non-symmetrical response, which is greater when turned ON than OFF, which is why in this case F1 better reflects the cortical response.

The NuDiva system displays the amplitude and phase in a real-time graph as a function of the spatial frequencies tested in the AV measurements, and as a function of the contrast levels tested in the CS measurements.

The same analysis was applied to two temporal frequencies close to the stimulation frequencies (fundamental) and their harmonics, but different from them. The aim of this second analysis was to obtain the electroencephalogram signal amplitude independent of the response to the visual stimulus. This amplitude constitutes what is considered "noise" while that measured at the stimulation frequency and its harmonics constitutes the "signal". A value of at least 3 in the signal-to-noise ratio was considered a fundamental requirement for the acceptance of recorded data.

AV or CS thresholds were estimated using an automated algorithm. In the case of AV, this algorithm plotted a linear fit of the amplitude data of the second harmonic as a function of spatial frequency, and in the case of SC, as a function of contrast. The AV and SC similars were obtained by extrapolating their linear fit function to zero amplitude. Examples of the analysis of both tests can be seen in figures 23 A and B.

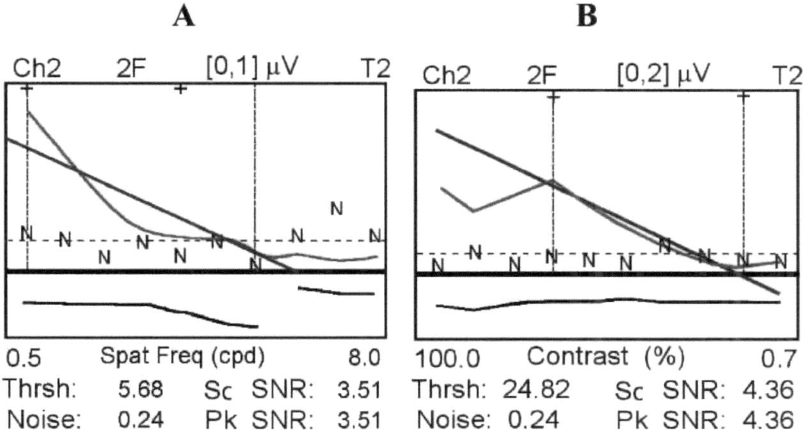

Fig. 22 - A. Example of the result obtained when measuring AV. Upper part of the graph. Ordinate: Amplitudes of the second harmonic of the PVCP scan for each of the 10 spatial frequencies represented on the abscissa, interpolated by a straight line. At each spatial frequency N indicates the EEG amplitude, whose average amplitude over the scan is represented by the dotted line. Lower part of the graph. Ordinate: phase of the response relative to the temporal pattern of stimulation - 0 to 180 degrees, abscissa, spatial frequencies.

B. Example of the result obtained when measuring the spatial SC of luminance at a spatial frequency of 2.0 cpg. Upper part of the graph. Ordinate: Amplitudes of the second harmonic of the Scanning PVCP for each of the 10 contrast levels represented on the abscissa. Lower part of the graph. Ordinate: phase of the response relative to the temporal pattern of stimulation, from 0 to 180 degrees. Abscissa: contrast levels.

Both results were obtained in baby number 3 born at term (table 3) at 3 months of age.

For a contrast scan to be considered valid by the experimenter, a signal-to-noise ratio (Pk SNR value in Figures 23 A and B) of 2:1 at peak amplitude for individual scans and 3:1 for averages was required.

As described above, there were two recording channels, one in each hemisphere, and a threshold was obtained on each of these channels. Three to twelve repetitions of scanning PVCPs (measurements) were carried out so that the three best AV and SC results with a good signal-to-noise ratio and constant phase were selected for the average. The final estimate of VA was expressed in cycles per degree (cpg) of visual angle, and of CS in percentage (%).

All the tests were carried out and analyzed by the same observer.

IV - Results

Visual acuity (VA) estimated by the threshold for resolving square grids with 80% contrast, expressed in cycles per degree, was assessed in premature babies (n=31) and those born at term (n=26), and in adults (n=9) (Figure 24). The data for premature infants is presented as a function of corrected age (months).

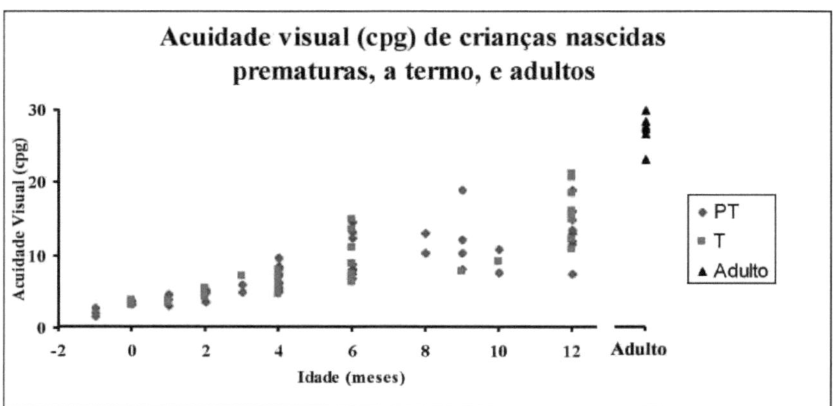

Fig. 24 - Visual acuity of all babies born prematurely (PT) and at term (T) assessed during the first year of life, as well as adults.

VA at the beginning of life is very low, in the order of 20/170 in the first month, and in premature infants it is even lower at the corrected age of -1 month (approximately 20/280). Over the course of development, VA showed a large increase (in cycles per degree of visual angle) in the first half of the year, followed by slower development in subsequent months, still not reaching the VA of adults by the end of the first year of life. These results include all the children evaluated, but given the small number of subjects at some ages, the study focused on a smaller number of ages at which it was possible to obtain a larger number of volunteers.

Thus, the VA results of children assessed at 4, 6 and 12 months of corrected age were selected for comparison between the groups of babies born prematurely and at term (figure 25).

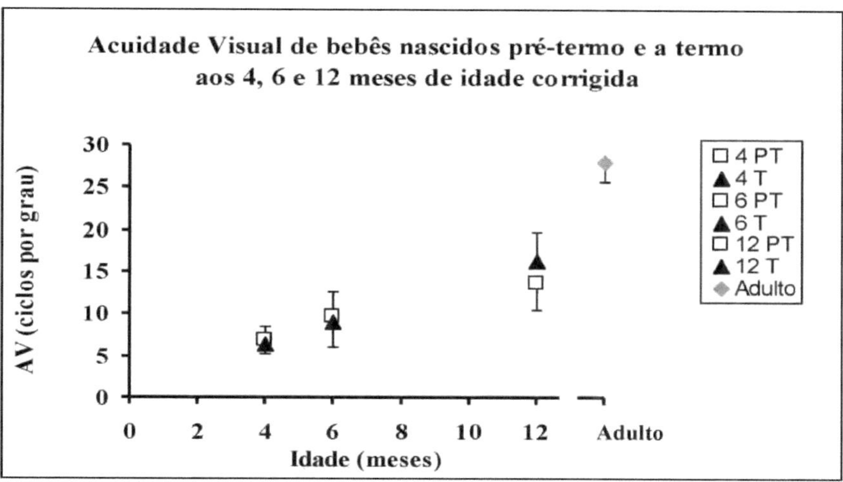

Fig. 25 - Mean and standard deviation of the visual acuities of babies born prematurely (PT) and at term (T) assessed at 4, 6 and 12 months of corrected age, as well as adults.

Preterm and full-term babies showed similar AV (cpg) results at all ages, with no statistically significant difference at any age (table 5).

Table 5 - Mean values, standard deviation (SD) and p* of the comparison of VA between premature and term babies

Age and subjects	Average	DP
4 months EN	7,01	1,54
4 months T	6,47	1,21
p-value - 4 months	0,462	
6 months EN	9,76	2,95
6 months EN	9,12	3,1
p-value - 6 months	0,414	
12 months EN	13,72	3,21
12 months EN	16,26	3,47
p-value - 12 months	0,212	

* Mann-Whitney rank sum T-test

No baby evaluated reached the average AV value of adults during the first year of life.

Threshold contrast (%) was determined in the same babies and in 14 adults at spatial frequencies of 0.2, 0.8, 2.0 and 4.0 cpg (Figures 26, 27, 28 and 29, respectively) and is shown as a function of age.

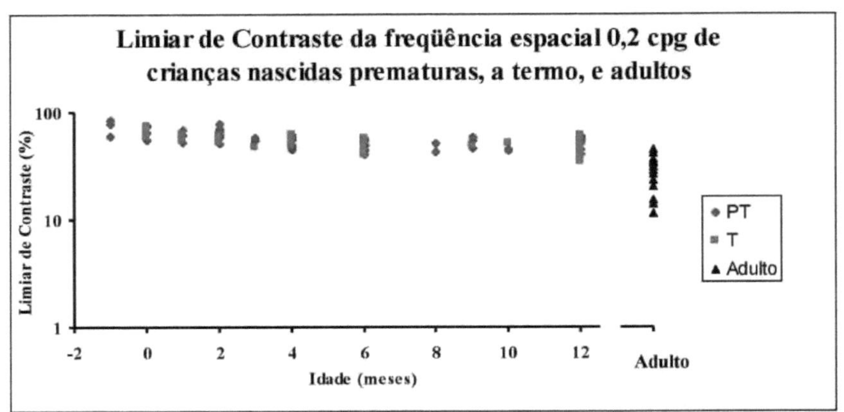
Limiar de Contraste da freqüência espacial 0,2 cpg de crianças nascidas prematuras, a termo, e adultos
Limiar de Contraste (%)
100
10
1
-2
0
2
4
6
8
10
12
Adulto
Idade (meses)
PT
T
Adulto

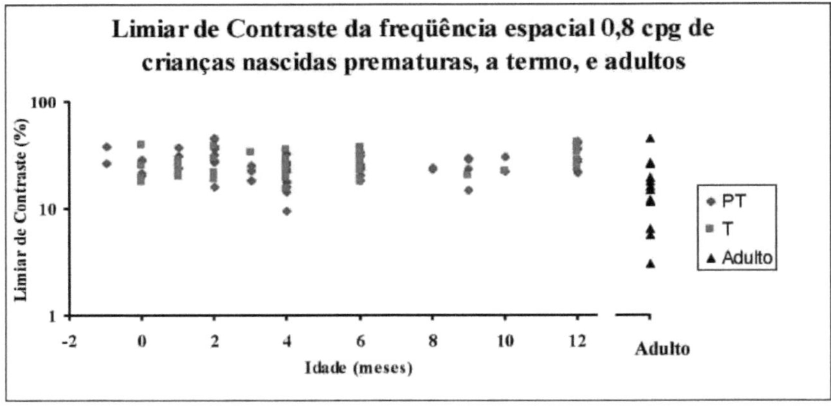
Limiar de Contraste da freqüência espacial 0,8 cpg de crianças nascidas prematuras, a termo, e adultos
Limiar de Contraste (%)
100
10
1
-2
0
2
4
6
8
10
12
Adulto
Idade (meses)
PT
T
Adulto

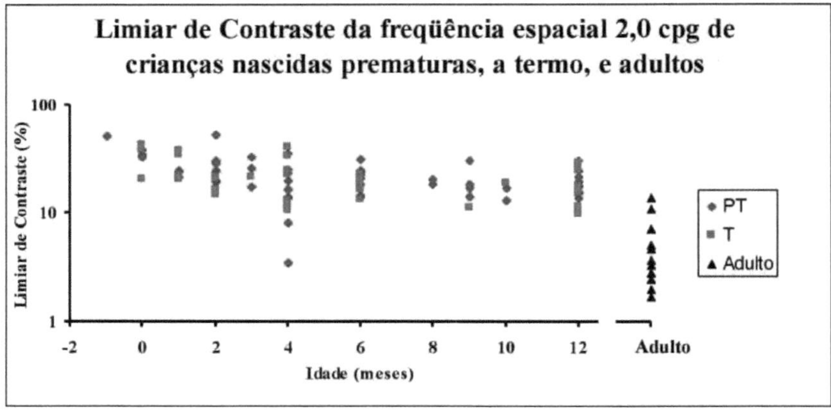
Limiar de Contraste da freqüência espacial 2,0 cpg de crianças nascidas prematuras, a termo, e adultos
Limiar de Contraste (%)
100
10
1
-2
0
2
4
6
8
10
12
Adulto
Idade (meses)
PT
T
Adulto

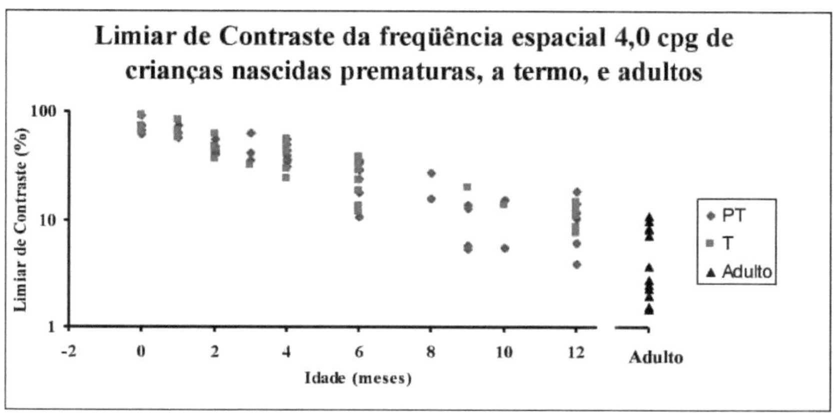

Fig. 26, 27, 28 and 29 - Contrast thresholds at spatial frequencies of 0.2, 0.8, 2.0 and 4.0 cpg, respectively, of all babies born prematurely (PT) and at term (T) assessed during the first year of life, as well as adults.

The data show different courses of contrast threshold development for the different spatial frequencies. Adult values are not reached in any of the spatial frequencies, even in the older babies (group assessed at 12 months corrected age). The 0.2 cpg spatial frequency, the lowest evaluated, showed the lowest development rate of all the frequencies. The 4.0 cpg spatial frequency, the highest evaluated, showed an exponential development curve. At 0.8 and 2.0 cpg, the two intermediate frequencies, development was faster in the first 3 or 4 months and slower after that.

Figure 30 brought together all the data contained in Figures 26, 27, 28 and 29, with the mean values for premature and term babies together at all the ages evaluated, but without including the standard deviation bars. The average CS thresholds for adults completed the figure.

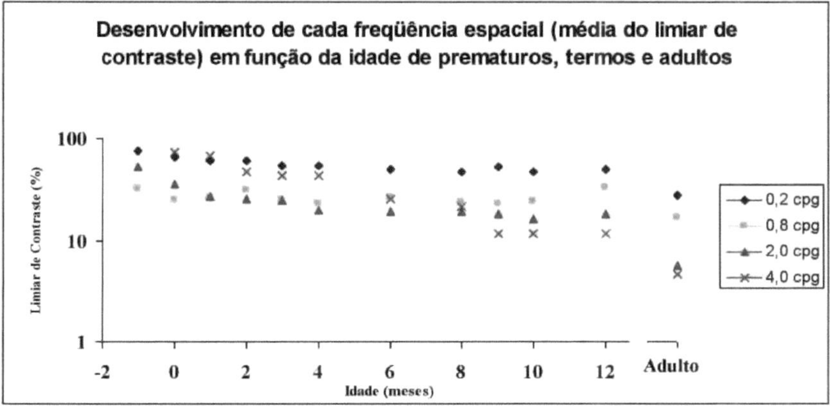

Fig. 30 - Average Contrast limares of the spatial frequencies 0.2, 0.8, 2.0 and 4.0 of babies born prematurely (PT) and at term (T) assessed during the first year of life, as well as adults.

The data confirms the different courses of development of each spatial frequency evaluated.

The contrast thresholds of the preterm and term infants assessed at 4, 6 and 12 months of corrected age (mean values for each age) were transformed into sensitivity values, and the CS function is presented as a function of spatial frequency, with AV values inserted to complete the CS curves, corresponding to the 80% contrast point (figures 31, 32 and 33, respectively).

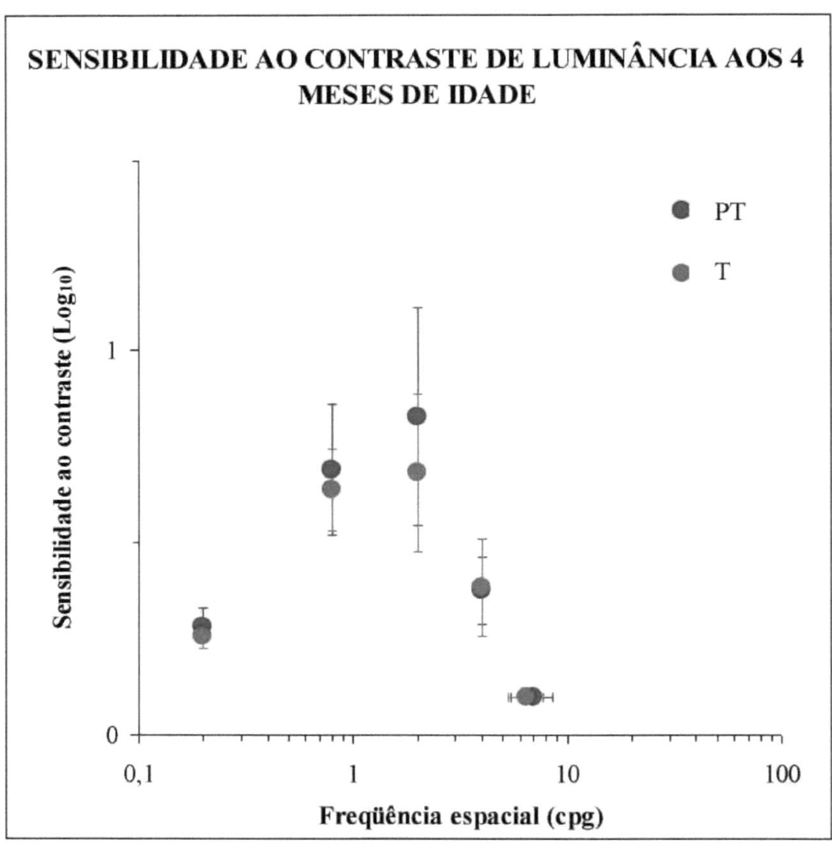

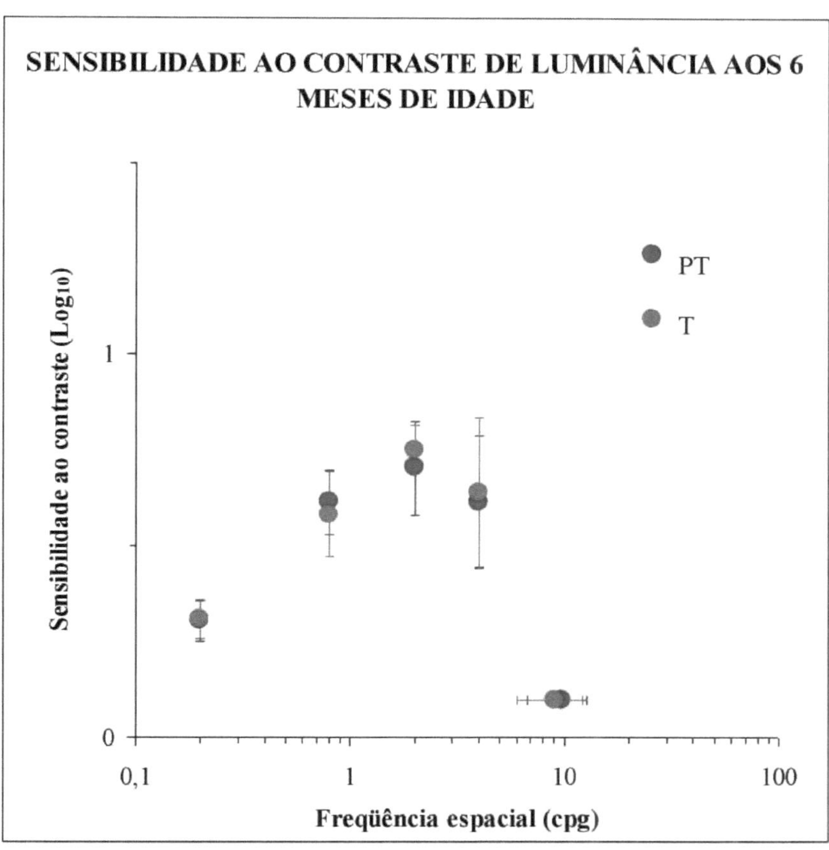
SENSIBILIDADE AO CONTRASTE DE LUMINÂNCIA AOS 6 MESES DE IDADE
Sensibilidade ao contraste (Log10)
1
0
PT
T
0,1
1
10
100
Freqüência espacial (cpg)

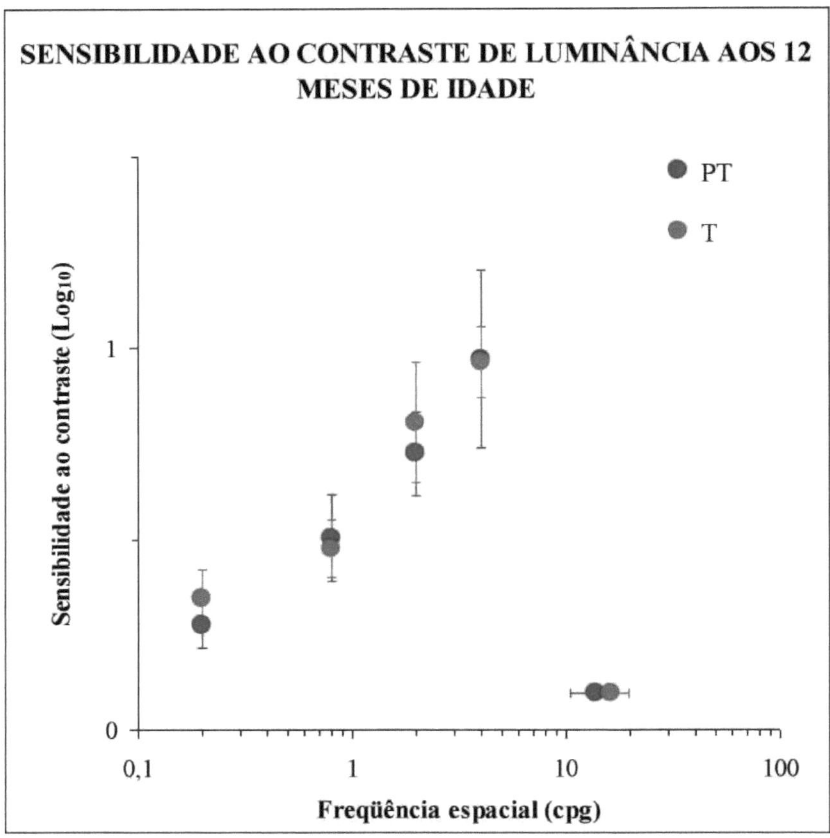

Fig. 31, 32 and 33 - Average contrast sensitivity and visual acuity of premature infants (PT) and term infants (T) at 4, 6 and 12 months of age, respectively.

Throughout development, the CS peak shifted to higher spatial frequencies. At 4 and 6 months, the peak occurred between the spatial frequencies 0.8 and 2.0 cpg. It then shifted to 4.0 at 12 months, when the CSF reached the same shape as this function in adults, but with a much lower CS.

The CS thresholds of preterm babies, as with VA, were not statistically different from those of full-term babies (table 6).

Table 6 - Mean values, standard deviation (SD) and p* of the comparison of CS between premature and term babies

Spatial frequency	0.2 cpg		0.8 cpg		2.0 cpg		4.0 cpg	
Age and subjects	**Mean**	**SD**	**Mean**	**SD**				
4 months EN	53,21	6,73	21,75	7,53	17,44	9,10	43,09	8,63
4 months T	55,73	4,05	23,78	5,87	22,91	10,04	43,06	11,20
p-value - 4 months	0,288		0,683		0,369		0,834	
6 months EN	50,16	6,06	24,69	4,87	20,48	5,77	25,76	8,39

6 months EN	49,87	5,54	26,89	6,74	17,93	2,65	25,12	10,37
p-value - 6 months	0,870		0,424		0,327		0,929	
12 months EN	53,34	7,02	32,34	8,07	19,49	5,19	11,93	5,24
12 months EN	45,94	8,16	33,88	5,57	16,66	6,43	11,15	2,28
p-value - 12 months	0,068		0,757		0,200		0,753	

* Mann-Whitney rank sum T-test

The data from Figures 3 1, 32 and 33 have been merged into Figure 34, including the adult data, to facilitate comparisons between ages.

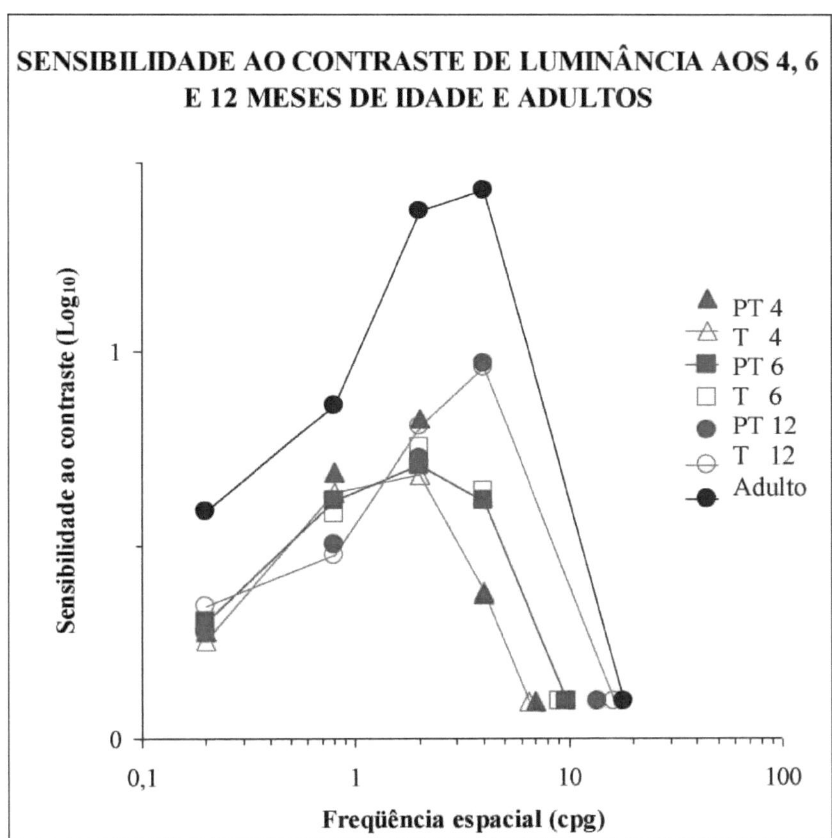

Fig. 34 - Average contrast sensitivity and visual acuity of premature infants (PT) and term infants (T) at 4, 6 and 12 months of age and of adults.

Unlike the AV results, the mean CS value for adults was reached by babies assessed at different ages at spatial frequencies of 0.8, 2.0 and 4.0 cpg.

One full-term baby and 2 premature babies, all assessed at 4 months, as well as another premature baby assessed at 9 months, reached the average value for adults (16.99%) at the spatial frequency 0.8 cpg, but the results of subsequent tests (at older ages) of the same babies showed lower results than the adults, showing the great modulation of sensitivity that occurs at this spatial frequency, which is the frequency of peak sensitivity at around 4 months of age.

A premature baby assessed at 4 months showed results comparable to the average for adults (16.99%) at a spatial frequency of 0.8 cpg, and also reached adult values (5.67%) at a frequency of 2.0 cpg.

The spatial frequency of 4.0 cpg also had only 1 baby born prematurely who reached the average for adults (4.66%) when assessed at 12 months corrected age.

Despite these individual cases, the thresholds covered a wide range of values, in which these examples are at the highest values. Thus, the average CS values of both premature and term infants for each age did not reach the adult values at any of the spatial frequencies evaluated.

AV and CS thresholds of the 4.0 cpg spatial frequency of preterm infants in the 4, 6 and 12 month corrected age groups were analyzed according to their Apgar score at the fifth minute of life, birth weight and gestational age. There was no correlation between the contrast threshold and the parameters Apgar score, birth weight and gestational age of the premature babies assessed at 4, 6 and 12 months of corrected age. Only the correlation between the contrast thresholds of the babies assessed at 12 months of corrected age and their gestational age values was high (0.7319), but this correlation can be attributed to the fact that more than half of this group of babies had the same gestational age value (32 weeks).

V - Conclusions and Discussion

The great development of the AV function during the first semester of life corroborates findings reported in previous studies (Dobson & Teller, 1978; Maurer et al., 1999; Norcia & Tyler, 1985; Salomao & Ventura, 1995; Schwartz, 2004; Sokol, 1978).

Like AV, CS also shows major changes during the development phase, modifying both the contrast thresholds of each spatial frequency and the shape of the CS curve, with the peak of sensitivity shifting to the higher frequencies, and with different developmental courses for each spatial frequency, confirming previous findings by Adams et al. (1992), Adams & Courage (1993), Atkinson, Braddick, & Moar (1977), Boothe et al. (1988) and Norcia, Tyler & Hamer (1990).

A discrepancy can be seen when comparing this work with that of Norcia, Tyler & Hamer (1990), in which 10-month-old babies reach adult thresholds at the lowest spatial frequencies.

In figure 34, which shows VA and CS data at 4, 6 and 12 months of age, in addition to the adults, the left arm of the curve shows overlapping data, forming a single function, up to 12 months, while after the peak, on the right side of the graph, the functions spread out in a fan and are approximately parallel as described by Norcia, Tyler & Hamer (1990). These authors described the existence of two processes in the development of AV and SC. Between 4 and 9 weeks all the spatial frequencies of the SC increased. After the ninth week, CS at low spatial frequencies remained constant while sensitivity increased systematically at high spatial frequencies. Our data seems to indicate the same developmental processes described by Norcia, Tyler & Hamer (1990). In the present data, this parallelism can be observed at a spatial frequency of 4.0 cpg, where CS increased from approximately 2.5% at 4 months, to 5.0% at 6 months, and to 10% at 12 months. Therefore, CS doubles in value from 4 to 6 months, and doubles again from 6 to 12 months, showing the great acceleration of the development process up to the sixth month of life. The adult value is approximately 40%, i.e. 4 times the CS value at 12 months (figure 35).

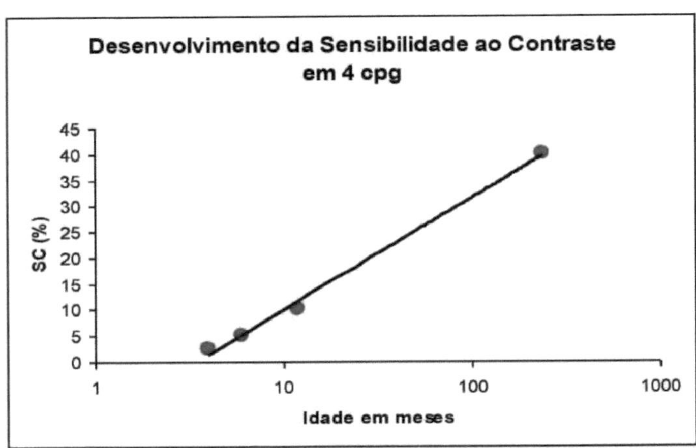

Fig. 35 - Development of contrast sensitivity for the spatial frequency of 4.0 cpg, showing that the increase in sensitivity is proportional to the logarithm of age.

Our data show that *there is* a significant difference between AV and SC thresholds at all spatial frequencies measured in adults and infants assessed during the first year of life. Our results follow the findings of Teller (1990), in which adult results are achieved after the third full year of life, Boothe et al. (1988), who showed spatial vision reaching adult levels between the third and fifth year of life, Montés-Micó & Ferrer-Blasco (2001), when children showed slow development of CSF between the third and seventh year of life, Jackson et al. (2003), who showed a slight increase in CBF as a function of age in children assessed between 7 and 13 years of age, and Adams & Courage (2002), who showed complete CBF maturation around the ninth year of life.

Measurements of the visual development of full-term and premature babies are an interesting tool for analyzing the function of visual experience. By comparing these two groups, babies of the same age but with different periods of visual experience are analyzed, and this could help to elucidate aspects of visual development that remain unknown.

In the present study, visual experience, studied in the way suggested above, did not affect the results, as no statistical differences were found between the VAs and CSs of term and premature babies, assessed using the scanning PVCP electrophysiological method. This result confirms our preliminary work (Oliveira et al., 2004) and also confirms the results of previous studies on differences in the VA of infants born at term and prematurely, assessed with reverse pattern PVCP (Rudduck & Harding, 1994; Kos-Pietro et al., 1997), scanning PVCP (Mazzitelli, 2002; Haro, 2003), and in the CS assessed psychophysically by Jackson et al. (2003). Another study showed similar results between preterm and term infants when assessed with the scanning PVCP, and superior results for preterm infants when assessed with the forced-choice preferential gaze technique (Baraldi et al., 1981). Mirabella et al. (2006), who also used the Scanning PVCP, found similar results for VA, CSF and vernier acuity for premature and term infants, with premature infants showing better amplitudes in contrast sensitivity and vernier acuity measurements.

On the other hand, some reports have disagreed, with lower results for premature infants. A study similar to that by Jackson et al. (2003), which assessed premature infants during adolescence using psychophysical methods, found lower results for premature infants in VA and CS (Lindqvist et al., 2007). Hammarrenger et al. (2007) found differences in the results of reverse pattern PVCP for one of the age groups evaluated, with lower results for premature infants for stimuli associated with magnocellular pathways.

The existence of perinatal complications makes the analysis more complex. Despite this, Van Hof-van J. & Mohn G. (1986) had demonstrated similar AV development in term and premature infants, even with minimal perinatal complications. On the other hand, premature infants with more severe complications evaluated by Jongmans et al. (1996), had alterations in VA and stereopsis, but their findings can be attributed to factors such as refractive error, strabismus, amblyopia, and damage to the post-chiasmatic region of the visual pathway. Other studies confirm findings of visual loss in patients born prematurely with some perinatal complication (Mash & Dobson, 1988), with poor visual attention and retrochiasmatic damage (Salomao et al., 2001), with altered neuropsychomotor development (Haro, 2003) or in the VA of premature infants with abnormal neurological examination (Morante et al. 1982). One study also reported better results in premature infants without alterations compared to those born at term, but restricted to the first few months of visual development, and which were later equalized between the groups of children (Haro, 2003).

As differences in VA and CS were assessed at the primary levels of the visual cortex, these results suggest that the primary visual processing of term and preterm babies is quite similar.

The present data suggests that the development of these two functions is very similar for both babies born at term and prematurely.

The data also suggest that there is no correlation between the AV and CS functions and the Apgar score, birth weight and gestational age of premature babies.

It is known that the visual system is dependent on experience, as Maurer et al. (1999) have shown. The present AV and SC data, in association with other spatial resolution studies (Baraldi et al., 1981) carried out on term and premature babies, suggest that visual experience does not affect the visual system's ability to resolve a spatial stimulus. This experience probably affects the synapses of the visual cortical areas that process visual information at higher levels in the visual associative cortex.

In conclusion, it seems that prematurity does not give babies better vision, but it does improve the processing and use of what they see. [2]

2 Data from some of these subjects at 3 and 10 months of age at spatial frequencies of 0.2 and 4.0 cpg were presented as a panel at the FeSBE Congress (Federation of Societies of Experimental Biology) in 2003 in Curitiba - PR, and the work was selected for oral presentation and awarded as a Finalist in the Young Researcher Competition - Michel Jamra Award 2003, by the Brazilian Society of Clinical Investigation - SBIC. As an award, the work received an invitation to be published in the *Brazilian Journal of Medical and Biological Research, which* was sent in 2003 and accepted in 2004. Preliminary results of the current work were presented as a panel in 2005 at the International Congress of ARVO (*The Association for Research in Vision and Ophthalmology*), held in Fort Lauderdale - FL - USA, and at the FeSBE Congress (Federation of Societies of Experimental Biology) also in 2005 in Aguas de Lindóia - SP, where he was awarded a Certificate of Merit by the organizing committee of the congress. In 2006 it was presented as a panel at the World Congress Ophthalmology in Sao Paulo - SP, and in 2007 it was again presented as a panel at the International Congress ARVO (*The Association for Research in Vision and Ophthalmology*), held in Fort Lauderdale - FL - USA.

VI - Bibliographical references

1. Adams, R. J., Mercer, M. E., Courage, M. L., & Vanhofvanduin, J. (1992). A New Technique to Measure Contrast Sensitivity in Human Infants. *Optometry and Vision Science, 69*, 440-446.

2. Adams, R. J. & Courage, M. L. (1993). Contrast Sensitivity in 24- Month-Olds and 36-Month-Olds As Assessed with the Contrast Sensitivity Card Procedure. *Optometry and Vision Science, 70*, 97-101.

3. Adams, R. J. & Courage, M. L. (2002). Using a single test to measure human contrast sensitivity from early childhood to maturity. *Vision Research, 42*, 1205-1210.

4. Allen, D., Banks, M. S., & Norcia, A. M. (1993). Does Chromatic Sensitivity Develop More Slowly Than Luminance Sensitivity. *Vision Research, 33,* 2553-2562.

5. Allen, D., Tyler, C. W., & Norcia, A. M. (1996). Development of grating acuity and contrast sensitivity in the central and peripheral visual field of the human infant. *Vision Research, 36*, 1945-1953.

6. Arippol, P. K. K., Salomao, S. R., & Belfort Jr., R. (2006). Computerized method for measuring visual acuity. *Arquivos Brasileiros de Oftalmologia, 69* (6), 907-914.

7. Atkinson, J., Braddick, O., & Braddick, F. (1974). Acuity and Contrast Sensitivity of Infant Vision. *Nature, 247,* 403-404.

8. Atkinson, J., Braddick, O., & Moar, K. (1977). Development of Contrast Sensitivity Over 1St 3 Months of Life in Human Infant. *Vision Research, 17,* 1037-1044.

9. Atkinson, J. & Braddick, O. (1989). Development of Basic Visual Fuctions. In Slater, A. & Bremner, G. (Eds.). Infant Development. Lawrence Erlbaum Associates.

10. Banks, M. S. & Salapatek, P.(1976). Contrast Sensitivity Function of the Infant Visual-System. *Vision Research, 16,* 867-869.

11. Baraldi, P., Ferrari, F., Fonda, S., & Penne, A. (1981). Vision in the Neonate (Full-Term and Premature) - Preliminary Result of the Application of Some Testing Methods. *Documenta Ophthalmologica, 51,* 101-112.

12. Beck, R. W., Moke, P. S., Turpin, A. H., Ferris III, F. L., SanGiovanni, J. P., Johnson, C. A., Birch, E. E., Chandler, D. L., Cox, T. A., Blair, R. C., & Kraker, R. T. (2003). A computerized method of visual acuity testing: Adaptation of the early treatment of diabetic retinopathy study testing protocol. *American Journal of Ophthalmology, 135*, 194-205.

13. Berezovsky, A., Salomao, S. R., Haro-Munoz, E., Ventura, D. F., Maffei, C. M. A., Hortelan,

L. R., Souza, E. C., & Bonomo, P. P. O. (1995). Monocular Visual Fields Measured in Eight Meridians by Double Arc Kinetic Perimetry in the First Year of Life. *Arquivos Brasileiros de Oftalmologia, 58,* 77-84.

14. Berezovsky, A., Moraes, N. S. B., Nusinowitz, S., & Salomao, S. R. (2003). Standard full-field electroretinography in healthy preterm infants. *Documenta Ophthalmologica, 107,* 243-249.

15. Bicas, H.E.A. (2002). Visual Acuity. Measurements and notations. *Brazilian Archives of Ophthalmology, 65* (3), 375-384

16. Birch, E. E. & Bane, M. C. (1991). Forced-Choice Preferential Looking Acuity of Children with Cortical Visual Impairment. *Developmental Medicine and Child Neurology, 33,* 722-729.

17. Birch, E. E. & O'Connor, A. R. (2001). Preterm birth and visual. *Development. Seminars in Neonatology, 6* (6), 487-497.

18. Bonotto, L. B., Moreira, A. T. R., & Carvalho, D. S. (2007). Prevalence of retinopathy of prematurity in premature infants seen in the period 1992-1999 in Joinville (SC): evaluation of associated risks - "screening". *Arquivos Brasileiros de Oftalmologia, 70,* 55-61.

19. Boothe, R. G., Kiorpes, L., Williams, R. A., & Teller, D. Y. (1988). Operant Measurements of Contrast Sensitivity in Infant Macaque Monkeys During Normal Development. *Vision Research, 28,* 387-396.

20. Bradley, A. & Freeman, R. D. (1982). Contrast Sensitivity in Children. *Vision Research, 22,* 953-959.

21. Campbell, F. W. & Robson, J. G. (1968). Application of Fourier Analysis to Visibility of Gratings. *Journal of Physiology-London, 197,* 551566.

22. Campbell, F. W. (1974). Contrast and Spatial Frequency. *Scientific American, 231,* 106-114.

23. Cinoto, R. W., Berezovsky, A., Belfort Jr., R., & Salomao, S. R. (2006). Comparison between self-reported quality of vision and visual acuity in a low-income elderly population in the city of Sao Paulo. *Arquivos Brasileiros de Oftalmologia, 69* (1), 17-22.

24. Cornsweet, T. N. (1970). Visual Perception. Academic Press.

25. Courage, M. L. & Adams, R. J. (1990). Visual-Acuity Assessment from Birth to 3 Years Using the Acuity Card Procedure - Cross-Sectional and Longitudinal Samples. *Optometry and Vision Science, 67,* 713-718.

26. da Costa, M. F., Salomao, S. R., Berezovsky, A., de Haro, F. M., & Ventura, D. F. (2004). Relationship between vision and motor impairment in children with spastic cerebral palsy: new

evidence from electrophysiology. *Behavioral Brain Research, 149,* 145-150.

27. Dambro, M. R. (2002). Griffith's 5-Minute Clinical Consult. Lippincott Ed.

28. de Faria, J. M. L., Katsumi, O., Arai, M., & Hirose, T. (1998). Objective measurement of contrast sensitivity function using contrast sweep visual evoked responses. *British Journal of Ophthalmology, 82,* 168-173.

29. Diamond, M. C. (2001). Response of the brain to enrichment. *Annals of the Brazilian Academy of Sciences, 73,* 21 1-220.

30. Dobkins, K. R. & Teller, D. Y. (1995). Infant contrast detectors are selective for direction of motion. *Vision Research, 36*, 281-294.

31. Dobkins, K. R., Lia, B., & Teller, D. Y. (1997). Infant color vision: Temporal contrast sensitivity functions for chromatically-defined stimuli in 3-month-olds. *Vision Research, 37*, 1-18.

32. Dobson, V. & Teller, D. Y. (1978). Visual acuity in human infants: a review and comparison of behavioral and electrophysiological studies. *Vision Research, 18,* 1469-1483.

33. Egyetem, P. O. & Klinika, S. N. (1999). Neonatal care of premature infants. *Orv Hetil, 140,* 161 1-1618.

34. Elliott, D. B. & Situ, P. (1998). Visual acuity versus letter contrast sensitivity in early cataract. *Vision Research, 38,* 2047-2052.

35. Hamer, R. D., Norcia, A. M., Tyler, C. W., & Hsuwinges, C. (1989). The Development of Monocular and Binocular Vep Acuity. *Vision Research, 29,* 397-408.

36. Hammerrenger, B., Roy, M. S., Ellenberg, D., Lambrosse, M., Orquin, J., Lippe, S., & Lepore, F. (2007). Developmental delay and magnocellular visual pathway function in very-low-birthweight preterm infants. *Developmental Medicine and Child Neurology, 49*, 28-33.

37. Harding, G. F. A., Odom, J. V., Spileers, W., & Spekreijse, H. (1996). Standard for visual evoked potentials 1995. *Vision Research, 36,* 3567-3572.

38. Haro, F. M. B. (2003). Development of grid-resolving visual acuity in premature infants during the first year of life: an electrophysiological study using scanning visual evoked potentials. *Doctoral thesis*. Faculty of Medicine, University of Sao Paulo, Sao Paulo.

39. Hart, W. M. (1992). Adler's physiology of the eye: clinical application. 9th ed. Mosby.

40. Harvey, E. M., Dobson, V., Luna, B., & Scher, M. S. (1997). Grating acuity and visual-field development in children with intraventricular hemorrhage. *Developmental Medicine and Child Neurology, 39,* 305-312.

41. Harwerth, R. S., Smith, E. L., Duncan, G. C., Crawford, M. L. J., & Vonnoorden, G. K. (1986). Multiple Sensitive Periods in the Development of the Primate Visual-System. *Science, 232,* 235-238.

42. Jackson, T. L., Ong, G. L., McIndoe, M. A., & Ripley, L. G. (2003). Monocular chromatic contrast threshold and achromatic contrast sensitivity in children born prematurely. *American Journal of Ophthalmology, 136,* 710-719.

43. Jasper, H. H. (1958). Report of the committee on methods of clinical examination in electroencephalography. *Electroencephalography and Clinical Neurophysiology, 10, 370-5.*

44. *Jongmans, M., Mercuri, E., Henderson, S., de Vries, L., Sonksen, P., & Dubowitz, L. (1996). Visual function of prematurely born children with and without perceptual-motor difficulties. Early Human Development, 45, 73-82.*

45. *Kelly, J. P., Borchert, K., & Teller, D. Y. (1997). The development of chromatic and achromatic contrast sensitivity in infancy as tested with the sweep VEP. Vision Research, 37, 2057-2072.*

46. *Kelly, J. P. & Chang, S. (2000). Development of chromatic and luminance detection contours using the sweep VEP. Vision Research, 40, 1887-1905.*

47. *Kolb, H., Fernandez, E., Nelson, R., & Jones, B. W. Retrieved January 10, 2007. Webvision - The Organization of the Retina and Visual System. University of Utah.*

http://webvision.med.utah.edu/

48. Kos-Pietro, S., Towle, V. L., Cakmur, R., & Spire, J. P. (1997). Maturation of human visual evoked potentials: 27 weeks conceptional age to 2 years. *Neuropediatrics, 28,* 3 18-323.

49. Lindqvist, S., Vik, T., Indredavik, M. S., & Brubakk, A. M. (2007). Visual acuity, contrast sensitivity, peripheral vision and refraction in low birthweight teenagers. *Acta Ophthalmologica Scandinavica, 85*, 157164.

50. Liu, C. Retrieved January 10, 2007. British Society for Refractive Surgery. Refractive surgery report: Visual performance.

http://www.bsrs2000.fsnet.co.uk/new page 13.htm

51. Lutty, G. A., Chan-Ling, T., Phelps, D. L., Adamis, A. P., Berns, K. Y., Chan, C. K., Cole, C. H., D'Amore, P. A., Das, A., Deng, W. T., Dobson, V., Flynn, J. T., Friedlander, M., Fulton, A., Good, W. V., Grant, M. A., Hansen, R., Hauswirth, W. W., & Robert, J. (2006). Proceedings of the Third International Symposium on Retinopathy of Prematurity: An uptade on ROP from the lab to the nursey (November 2003, Anaheim, California). *Molecular Vision,* 12, 532-580.

52. Mash, C. & Dobson, V. (1998). Long-term reliability and predictive validity of the teller acuity

card procedure. *Vision Research, 38,* 619-626.

53. Maurer, D., Lewis, T. L., Brent, H. P., & Levin, A. V. (1999). Rapid improvement in the acuity of infants after visual input. *Science, 286*, 108-110.

54. Mayer, D. L. & Dobson, V. (1982). Visual acuity development in infants and young children as assessed by operant preferential looking. *Vision Research, 22*, 1 141-1 151.

55. Mayer, D. L., Beiser, A. S., Warner, A. F., Pratt, E. M., Raye, K. N., & Lang, J. N. (1995). Monocular acuity norms for the Teller Acuity Cards between ages one month and four years. *Investigative Ophthalmology & Visual Science, 36,* 671-685.

56. Mazzitelli, C. (2002). Neuromotor development of premature infants included in an early stimulation program. *Master's dissertation.* Institute of Psychology, University of Sao Paulo, Sao Paulo.

57. McDonald, M. A., Dobson, V., Sebris, S. L., Baitch, L., Varner, D., & Teller, D. Y. (1985). The acuity card procedure: A rapid test of infant acuity. *Investigative Ophthalmology & Visual Science, 26,* 1 158-1 162.

58. Mills, M. D. (1999). The Eye in Childhood. *American Family Physician, 60*, 907-918.

59. Mirabella, G., Kjaer, P. K., Norcia, A. M., Good, W. V., & Madan, A. (2006). Visual Development in Very Low Birth Weight Infants. *Pediatric Research, 60*, 1 -5.

60. Montés-Micó, R. & Ferrer-Blasco, T. (2001). Contrast sensitivity function in children: normalized notation for the assessment and diagnosis of diseases. *Documenta Ophthalmologica, 103,* 175-1 86.

61. Morante, A., Dubowitz, L. M., Leven, M., & Dubowitz, V. (1982). The development of visual function in normal and neurologically abnormal preterm and fullterm infants. *Developmental Medicine and Child Neurology, 24,* 771-784.

62. Moskowitz, A. & Sokol, S. (1980). Spatial and Temporal Interaction of Pattern-Evoked Cortical Potentials in Human Infants. *Vision Research, 20,* 699-707.

63. Moutquin, J. M. (2003). Classification and heterogeneity of preterm birth. *Bjog-An International Journal of Obstetrics and Gynaecology, 110,* 30-33.

64. Norcia, A. M. & Manny, R. E. (2003). Development of Vision in Infancy. In: Kaufman, P. L. & Alm, A. Adler's Physiology of the eye. Clinical Application. (10 ed.) Mosby.

65. Norcia, A. M. & Tyler, C. W. (1985). Spatial frequency sweep VEP: visual acuity during the first year of life. *Vision Research, 25,* 13991408.

66. Norcia, A. M., Tyler, C. W., Hamer, R. D., & Wesemann, W. (1989). Measurement of Spatial Contrast Sensitivity with the Swept Contrast Vep. *Vision Research, 29,* 627-637.

67. Norcia, A. M., Tyler, C. W., & Hamer, R. D. (1990). Development of contrast sensitivity in the human infant. *Vision Research, 30,* 1475-1486.

68. Odom, J. V. (2003). Functional vision: assessment and outcome. *Visual Impairment Research, 5,* 1 13-1 14.

69. Odom, J. V., Bach, M., Barber, C., Brigell, M., Marmor, M. F., Tormene, A. P., Holder, G. E., & Vaegan (2004). Visual evoked potentials standard. *Documenta Ophthalmologica, 108*, 1 15-123.

70. Ohzawa, I. Retrieved January 10, 2007. Make Your Own Campbell-Robson Contrast Sensitivity Chart **http://cobalt056.bpe.es.osaka-u.ac.jp/ohzawa- lab/izumi/CSF/A JG RobsonCSFchart.html**

71. Oliveira, A. G. F., Costa, M. F., de Souza, J. M., & Ventura, D. F. (2004). Contrast sensitivity threshold measured by sweep-visual evoked potential in term and preterm infants at 3 and 10 months of age. *Brazilian Journal of Medical and Biological Research, 37,* 1389-1396.

72. Ornelas, S. L., Xavier, C. C., & Colosimo, E. A. (2002). Growth of preterm newborns. *Jornal de Pediatria, 78* (3), 230236.

73. Parmelee, A. H. (1975). Neurophysiological and Behavioral Organization of Premature-Infants in 1St Months of Life. *Biological Psychiatry, 10,* 501-512.

74. Peterzell, D. H. & Norcia, A. M. (1997). Spatial frequency masking with the sweep-VEP. *Vision Research, 37,* 2349-2359.

75. Pike, M. G., Holmstrom, G., de Vries, L. S., Pennock, J. M., Drew, K. J., Sonksen, P. M., & Dubowitz, L. M. S. (1994). Patterns of visual impairment associated with lesions of the preterm infant brain. *Developmental Medicine and Child Neurology, 36,* 849-862.

76. Pirchio, M., Spinelli, D., Fiorentini, A., & Maffei, L. (1978). Infant Contrast Sensitivity Evaluated by Evoked-Potentials. *Brain Research, 141,* 179-184.

77. Porciatti, V., Ciavarella, P., Ghiggi, M. R., D'Angelo, V., Padovano, S., Grifa, M., & Moretti, G. (1999). Losses of hemifield contrast sensitivity in patients with pituitary adenoma and normal visual acuity and visual field. *Clinical Neurophysiology, 110,* 876-886.

78. Rades, E., Bittar, R. E., & Zugaib, M. (2004). Direct Determinants of Elective Premature Delivery and Neonatal Outcomes. *Brazilian Journal of Gynecology and Obstetrics, 26* (8), 655-662.

79. Rasengane, T. A., Allen, D., & Manny, R. E. (1997). Development of temporal contrast

sensitivity in human infants. *Vision Research, 37,* 1747-1754.

80. Regal, D. M. (1981). Development of critical flicker frequency in human infants. *Vision Research, 21,* 549-555.

81. Rodrigues, A. R., Botelho de Souza, C. R., Braga, A. M., Rodrigues, P. S. S., Silveira, A. T., Damin, E. T. B., Côrtes, M. I. T., Castro, A. J. O., Mello, G. A., Vieira, J. L. F., Pinheiro, M. C. N., Ventura, D. F., & Silveira, L. C. L. (2007). Mercury toxicity: contrast sensitivity and color discrimination of subjects exposed to mercury. *Brazilian Journal of Medical and Biological Research, 40*, 415-424.

82. Rudduck, G. A. & Harding, G. F. A. (1994). Visual Electrophysiology to Achromatic and Chromatic Stimuli in Premature and Full-Term Infants. *International Journal of Psychophysiology, 16,* 209-218.

83. Salomao, S. R. & Ventura, D. F. (1995). Large-Sample Population Age Norms for Visual Acuities Obtained with Vistech-Teller Acuity Cards. *Investigative Ophthalmology & Visual Science, 36,* 657-670.

84. Salomao, S. R., Berezovsky, A., De Haro, F. M. B., Goldchmit, M., & Ventura, D. F. (2001). Grating acuity deficit in preterm infants with cortical visual impairment. *Investigative Ophthalmology & Visual Science, 42,* S845.

85. Santos, N. A. & Simas, M. L. B. (2001). Contrast Sensitivity Function. *Psicologia: Reflexão e Critica, 14,* 589-597.

86. Schwartz, S. H. (2004). Visual perception: a clinical orientation. (3ed.) McGraw-Hill Companies.

87. Shannon, E., Skoczenski, A. M., & Banks, M. S. (1996). Retinal illuminance and contrast sensitivity in human infants. *Vision Research, 36,* 67-76.

88. Shapley, R., Kaplan, E., & Purpura, K. (1993). Contrast sensitivity and light adaptation in photoreceptors or in the retinal network. 5, 103-1 17. In Shapley, R. and Lam, D. M-K. Contrast Sensitivity Proceedings of the Retinal Research Foundation Symposia. MIT Press.

89. Slater, A. (1989). Visual Development. In Slater, A. & Bremner, G. (Eds.). Infant Development. Lawrence Erlbaum Associates.

90. Sokol, S. (1978). Measurement of Infant Visual-Acuity from Pattern Reversal Evoked-Potentials. *Vision Research, 18,* 33-39.

91. Souza, G. D., Gomes, B. D., Saito, C. A., Silveira, L. C. L., & da Silva Filho, M. (2006). Human Achromatic Spatial Contrast Sensitivity Measured With Transient Visual Evoked Cortical Potential:

Comparison With Psychophysics Measurements. *Investigative Ophthalmology & Visual Science, 47,* E-Abstract 5370.

92. Spallicci, M. D. B., Chiea, M. A., Albuquerque, P. B., Bittar, R. E., & Zugaib, M. (2000). Study of some maternal variables related to prematurity at the University Hospital of the University of Sao Paulo. *Revista Mèdica do Hospital Universitàrio - USP, 10* (1), 19-23.

93. StJohn, R. (1997). Contrast detection and orientation discrimination thresholds associated with meridional amblyopia. *Vision Research, 37,* 1451-1457.

94. Teller, D. Y. (1990). The Development of Visual Function in infants. In Cohen, B. & Bodis-Wollner, L.(Eds.). Vision and the Brain. Raven Press.

95. Teller, D. Y. (1997). First Glances: The Vision of Infants. The Friendwald Lecture. *Investigative Ophthalmology & Visual Science, 38* (11), 2183-2203.

96. Teller, D. Y. (1998). Spatial and temporal aspects of infant color vision. *Vision Research, 38,* 3275-3282.

97. Van Hof-van Duin, J. & Mohn, G. (1986). The Development of Visual Acuity in Normal Fullterm and Preterm Infants. *Vision Research, 26* (6), 909-916.

98. Ventura, D. F., Quiros, P., Carelli, V., Salomao, S. R., Gualtieri, M., Oliveira, A. G. F., Costa, M. F., Berezovsky, A., Sadun, F., & Sadun, A. A. (2005). Chromatic and luminance contrast sensitivities of carriers of 1 1778 Leber's Hereditary Optic Neuropathy (LHON) from a giant pedigree in Brazil. *Investigative Ophthalmology & Visual Science, 46,* 4809-4814.

99. Ventura, D. F., Simoes, A. L., Tomaz, S., Costa, M. F., Lago, M., Costa, M. T. V., Pereira, L. H. M. C., Souza, J. M., Faria, M. A. M., & Silveira, L. C. L. (2005). Color vision and contrast sensitivity losses of mercury intoxicated industry workers in Brazil. *Environmental Toxicology and Pharmacology, 19,* 523-529.

100. Ventura, D. F. Retrieved January 10, 2007. Vision Laboratory: Psychophysics and Clinical Visual Electrophysiology. Institute of Psychology, University of Sao Paulo.

http://www.ip.usp.br/laboratorios/visual/

101. World Health Organization (WHO) (1970). The prevention of perinatal mortality and morbidity. 457.

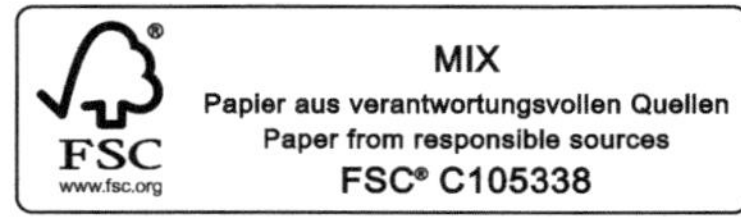

Printed by Books on Demand GmbH, Norderstedt / Germany